CICELY

The Story of a Doctor

To John & Harriet

with love from Ann

Ann Dally

Christmas 1968

Helen!

See page 30

" 95

CICELY

The Story of a Doctor

by

ANN DALLY

LONDON
VICTOR GOLLANCZ LTD
1968

575 00096 1

Printed in Great Britain by
The Camelot Press Ltd., London and Southampton

INTRODUCTION

Dr Cicely Williams is unusual and outstanding. She became well known as the first person to write a full description of the deadly disease *kwashiorkor* and to discover its true nature. We now know that this disease, which is entirely preventable, kills more children than any other disease in the world. Her work on this subject made her famous in the 1930s. It is described in this book, together with the highly individual way in which she made her discovery.

But nowadays Dr Williams is even better known because she has revolutionised ideas of child care in the tropics and has started a whole new way of thinking about the subject. This has come about through the events of her life and through her unusual personality. She is essentially an innovator, and has always shown unusual persistence and devotion in her work, dominated by feelings for humanity and by marked intellectual curiosity. She approached every problem with compassion and an open mind. For instance, she was as ready to learn from witch doctors as from up-to-date drugs, and many of her patients benefited as a result.

Dr Williams, now in her seventies, is retired. The American Medical Association recently awarded her their Joseph Goldberger Award for outstanding contributions to clinical nutrition. This is the latest of her many awards and honours.

Many people who know Cicely Williams, either personally or by repute, wonder how she came to be what she is and how it was that an old landowning family, steeped in traditions and responsibilities, could produce a daughter so remarkable.

This book attempts to show how it happened.

TO JEAN

CHAPTER I

She hurried out to meet him as though she had been waiting.

"How do you do? I'm Cicely Williams. I'm so relieved that you've come."

She was framed in the doorway of the clinic house, a low hut with a wattle roof. He recognised her at once. She had been on the ship coming out to West Africa six weeks ago. Tallish, erect and slender, with a rather large nose, a firm chin, and skin that was strikingly white, even for a European. He remembered that he had thought her graceful and gawky, and also serious. Yet she had danced an apache dance with abandon at the fancy dress ball the night before they docked.

They shook hands. "I'm John Ferrers."

"I'm so relieved you've come," she repeated. "The patient's inside. Have you brought the Petrie dishes?"

"Petrie dishes? I don't understand."

"Aren't you the doctor from the hospital at Korle Bu?" she asked suspiciously.

"No. I'm a District Commissioner. I've come to take you to a tennis tournament." The words flowed incongruously.

He had heard that she was humorous and attractive but intense. The Director of Medical Services on the Gold Coast had heard about her too, and had asked John to drive her to the club.

"Tennis? Good God, yes, I forgot. There is a bit of an emergency here this afternoon. I thought the hospital at Korle Bu might send someone."

"What's the trouble?"

"A boy with diphtheria."

"Diphtheria?" He was astonished. "Surely that's impossible. There isn't any in the Gold Coast. At least, that's what we were told in our First Aid lectures."

"That's what I was told too," she said ruefully. "I rang up Medical H.Q. and asked them for some anti-diphtheria serum. I got the impression they thought I was mad."

"Are you sure it's diphtheria?"

"I can't be absolutely certain until the lab. has identified it, but that's what it looks like. Luckily the child isn't seriously ill. They aren't always, you know. All the same, I bet you ninety-nine to one it's diphtheria, and if so he needs an injection of anti-diphtheria serum at once."

"Can you be so certain?" He was thinking how new she was to the job, to Africa and its many unique problems, and also to Africans, who are in many ways so different from other people.

"You can't mistake it once you really know it. Also it *looks* like diphtheria down the microscope. Medical H.Q. seem to be quite excited and said they would see if they have any serum. They'll ring back any minute now."

An unusual woman, he thought, particularly in the Gold Coast, where European women were few, and allowed to accompany their husbands only on condition that they left their children behind. Their babies were never born in the "White Man's Grave", where yellow fever was common and deadly. Most wives chose to stay away, and found separation tolerable because the men went home every eighteen months. To compensate for the discomforts and dangers of West Africa they had a week's leave for every month of service. A few women chose to travel with their husbands. There were also some in the Government Service, all unmarried. Dr Williams was one of these.

His throat felt dry, for it was December, the season when the Harmattan blows, the dusty trade wind that dries up the timber and vegetation as well as one's own throat and covers everything with a red dust.

A group of African mothers with babies and young children stood just inside the door, chatting. They smiled and moved aside. One scurried away through the red dust with her baby on her back, its small head wobbling. Ferrers hesitated briefly, then greeted them in their own language. The women smiled and seemed pleased.

"You speak wonderful Ga," said Cicely, admiringly.

He grinned. "I've just passed the exam."

"Some English people seem to think that if you shout loudly enough in English everyone will understand. But however much one wants to talk it's a difficult language to learn."

"The languages here are mostly tone languages, which makes them difficult for Europeans. It has taken me four years to talk Ga."

The telephone rang and she hurried into the inner room. Through the door Ferrers could see a boy of about ten with his mother beside him. Presumably he was the case of diphtheria. Cicely greeted them in friendly English, though they obviously did not understand. John kept a wary distance and moved to the other end of the hut, where a cheerful nurse was sorting medicine bottles. Her clean white coat gleamed against her shiny black cheeks and she was singing quietly. He wondered whether to try a conversation. Unless you got it exactly right, you could produce the most peculiar reactions in Africans by trying to speak their languages. Then it occurred to him that she probably spoke English.

"Finished for the day?"

She smiled and showed her straight white teeth.

"Yessir, but Miss Doctor Williams, she arrange bed in hospital for boy with throat sickness. She very good doctor, take very good care. She know many things."

A woman came through the door with a baby on her back and twin toddlers at her side. The twins looked apathetic and moved slowly, with large bellies, peeling skins and a faint faded reddish tinge to their hair. The mother spoke to the nurse in a language John did not understand, and the nurse handed her a bottle and a spoon. Just then Cicely came out through the door and smiled at the mother.

"Has this mother everything she needs?" she asked the nurse.

"Yes, doctor."

"And she understands that she must bring the twins again

in three days? Three days." She held up three fingers to the mother.

The nurse spoke briefly in the mother's language and also held up three fingers. "Yes, doctor. She understand and say thank you."

Cicely stroked the babies' heads. "Korle Bu say they've found some serum but it was out of date in 1918."

"Good God. Eleven years ago. Will it do?"

"No. Too risky. We'll have to do without."

"What else are you going to do?" He was thinking of her host, waiting in Accra.

"I've arranged for the child to be taken to hospital and now I'm ready to come with you. I've seen seventy patients since lunch and I've had enough."

"Those twins," she said as they walked across the dusty compound towards the car. "Did you notice anything odd about them?"

"They don't look very well, do they?" John said. "And their hair is peculiar."

"Exactly. It's a mysterious disease. No one seems to know anything about it and it's not in the textbooks."

"So?" asked John, probing again.

"So I'm going to find out about it," said Cicely, decisively.

He closed the door of the old Ford and climbed into the driver's seat beside her.

"The sun doesn't seem to worry you, but you can easily get sunstroke out here. I know you're a doctor but you've only just come out from England, haven't you?"

She smiled. "I've only been here for six weeks, but I was born and brought up in the tropics so I'm used to the sun. It can be hot in Jamaica, where I come from."

"You're lucky to stand it so well. I find the sun murderous." He eased the car forward along the dusty red road that led to the capital.

"We've met before, I think," she said. "Briefly."

"Yes. You looked charming at that party."

She ignored the compliment. "I remember which one you

were. I've been trying to place you. You were the Roman Senator hanging upside down from a pillar and gibbering like a monkey."

"I should have preferred being the man dressed as a life-saver who was whirling you round by the heels."

"It was dreadful. I never felt so giddy in my life. Not very good behaviour for a new medical officer!"

"Did your relations mind your coming out here?" asked John. "Even if you are used to the tropics it must be very different here from Jamaica."

"My family were rather shocked. They told me that people only come out here if they have to and that you generally pack your goods in your coffin when you come. But once I get a feeling about what I must do, I go ahead and do it. Now I feel that it's part of my destiny. There's so much work to be done here. Do you know that more than half the children die before they grow up? And that's not counting the ones who die at birth. Even the diseases they die of aren't the ones that we are taught about in England."

"Look." He pointed towards the sea shining red in the distance. "There's the castle of Christiansborg."

"It's wonderful," she said, looking at the big castle on the shore, "especially with the sun shining on it like that."

"It reminds me of Asameni."

"Who's he?"

"He was a splendid character, a local chief who captured the castle at the end of the seventeenth century. He used to dress up in the Danish Governor's uniform and fire continuous salutes in his own honour. Later on the castle fell on evil days. At one time it was even used as a lunatic asylum. But now it's magnificent again and the Governor lives there. He'll invite you to a party some time."

"Are all the castles on the Coast like that?"

"No. This one is still used, although of course there are masses of them, all along the coast. They were built as collecting points for slaves, and pretty well every coastal village seems to have one. They are all sizes and shapes, some small and insignificant, some enormous like Christiansborg or Cape Coast. Most of them are empty now except for dogs and chickens and children playing. Sometimes you may find one room used as a post office, and a few we use as Government rest houses."

"A curious legacy of the slave trade," said Cicely, "and I've already noticed another result of it. The depopulation of the country is terrible. I came from Kumasi to Accra by rail the other day, and the forests were scarcely inhabited at all."

"From the number of babies they have," he said, "you'd imagine the place would be overpopulated. The women all want babies all the time."

"But think what a lot of them die," she said. "Still, it's true what you said about their wanting babies. The women will do anything if they think it will lead to having more children. Their prestige seems to depend on their fertility really more than it depends on the number of children who actually survive."

"You're very perceptive. It took me three years to learn that."

She smiled. "I feel very much at home already."

"Look," said John Ferrers, pointing across the tennis court towards a lean, active man who had just won a game with a spectacular half volley. "There's your boss and Lord High Executioner, Dr Henry O'Hara May, Director of Medical Services in the Gold Coast."

"I thought he'd be an old buffer," exclaimed Cicely.

"He can't be all that young. He's been here for years and years. I'll have to make myself scarce when he comes off the court. He more or less told me so when he asked me to collect you."

"He sounds a bit of an autocrat," she said, as Dr O'Hara May sliced again at the ball, well below the level of the net. Half-volleys were obviously his speciality.

"Not really," John laughed. "His boys like him well enough. He's a bit unusual, that's all. Believes in calling a spade a spade. I'm told that he always gives the appearance of doing nothing at all and not caring about anything. But in fact he's doing first-class work."

"People like that appeal to me."

O'Hara May won the match with three half-volleys placed cunningly to catch his opponent unawares, and shook hands warmly with the much younger man he had defeated. Then, still smiling, he walked quickly towards John and Cicely.

"You must be Dr Williams. Marvellous to see you." He flung out both his arms in a curious bear-like attitude.

"How do you do?" Cicely said diffidently, with a sudden irrational desire to curtsey. As a little girl she had been taught to curtsey to grown-up strangers, and the desire came back when she was nervous, sometimes in inappropriate circumstances. Both her parents had been particular about politeness.

Instead of shaking hands he put his arm round her shoulders. "You and I are going for a little walk," he said. "There are lots of things I want to talk to you about. Goodbye, Ferrers. Thanks for your help. I'm sure you enjoyed Cicely's company as much as I'm going to."

"Goodbye, sir. Yes, sir," John answered, respectful yet grinning. He gave Cicely a half-wink and left.

"I gather you've saddled us with a case of diphtheria," said Dr O'Hara May as he steered her away from the crowd. "Let me congratulate you on your powers of diagnosis—though I ought to slay you for introducing new diseases into this disease-ridden country."

"Oh!" She was taken aback. "How did you know? It only happened this afternoon."

"The Senior Pathologist at Korle Bu has already examined your swab, and he agrees with your diagnosis. I have little doubt that, unfortunately, diphtheria, a disease hitherto unknown in this country and therefore never thought of except by the most exceptional and outstanding doctors, is now with us, and we shall have to gear our entire medical services towards dealing with the problem."

She couldn't tell whether he was joking or serious, and this made her nervous.

"I'm sorry."

"Sorry?" he roared. "What on earth are you apologising about? Good God, woman, you're brilliant. And why did you look so scared when I said hello? You're not really scared. You're as tough as nails underneath, aren't you? I don't know how you managed to get yourself trained, but I'm sure it must have been a struggle. What's more, your medical experience since you qualified has been first-rate. How did you manage it?"

Cicely, suddenly nervous no longer, found it easy to tell him something of her background, and of the combination of events which had brought her to the Gold Coast.

People who knew her later in her life sometimes thought that she must have had a vocation to go to Africa. Her total absorption with her work there, the sureness of her step and the way in which she always seemed to know what to do next, suggested a culmination of years of hopes and intentions. But this was not so. Cicely had no early vocation, and no desire to go to Africa or to work anywhere other than in England.

She went abroad in desperation, almost by mistake, because she couldn't get a job in England. Qualifying as a doctor had been hard, for women were still on the fringe of the profession, and even when she had had several years' experience in British hospitals no one seemed to need her. In the end she got fed up and swore that she would take whatever job was offered, and so she went to Greece and looked after refugees.

In Greece she learnt how to control malaria, and began to understand the importance of food in health and disease. She discovered that the local cure for a tarantula bite was to get forty virgins to spit in your mouth. She saw children sick and dying of diseases that no one had yet identified, let alone cured. At the end of it all she knew that the only life she wanted was working abroad.

Cicely had been born in Jamaica, the daughter of Rowland Williams, a well-known landowner there. Like other landed families in Jamaica, the Williamses had lost their wealth when slavery was abolished on the island in 1836. When Cicely was a child her parents were living at Kew Park, a large but impoverished estate which provided work for many devoted coloured servants and estate workers. Some had been there for more than half a century. Both Rowland and his wife were of unusually even temperament, and Kew Park, in spite of its finances, was a happy place.

The children lived an open air life and were devoted to their home and parents. But though they felt immensely secure, their father knew that there could be no question of independent means for them. Rowland was a thoughtful, cheerful, far-sighted man, and he was aware that, to young people of their background and position at that time, having no money was a serious matter.

Soon after Queen Victoria died he studied his daughters carefully, and decided that the oldest and the youngest were straightforward. They would marry and would never have to earn their living. But there was something about nine-year-old Cicely that roused her father's old forgotten joys, his painful regrets and his lost ambitions. Of all his children she was the one who stood out in his feelings. And she adored him.

"You'll never find a husband, my dear. You had better go to Oxford when you are old enough, and learn to be a lady doctor."

"Yes, Father," the child replied, docile and not apparently much interested.

Cicely, who was supposed to be a delicate child, always believed that she only thought of becoming a doctor because her father had suggested it. It was certainly an unusual suggestion. In Edwardian times it was very much not the custom for daughters of Jamaican landowners, or indeed of landowners anywhere, to go to university or to study medicine, and women doctors were few and still regarded as oddities. For a while she thought quite seriously about what her father had said, but then gradually forgot it. For years her chief interests were in the ordinary life of upper-class Jamaica, riding and tennis and dances, in between lessons from a governess until she was twelve, when she first went to England to school. Her father continued to mention Oxford from time to time. Cicely felt that she might like to study English or History there one day, but when she was old enough to go there was not enough money to send her. So while her three brothers finished their education she stayed at home, content, as always, with tennis, riding, gardening and housekeeping. She taught for a period in a Montessori school, an experience which was of great value in her later career.

In spite of the strange fire that burned in her, Cicely fitted in quietly with whatever life offered. She still thought of Oxford sometimes, but in 1914 it seemed further away than ever. Yet the war revived her childhood interest in healing, and First Aid and Home Nursing classes brought back the old idea of studying medicine. She discovered that once she knew how to do something she no longer felt squeamish about it. Soon she was dealing with minor accidents and sickness among her father's employees and, to Rowland Williams' great joy, announced that if and when she could go to university she would study medicine.

On Easter Day, 1916, Rowland Williams died. After this Cicely became increasingly impatient to begin her studies. But before anything definite could be arranged all passports for women and children to travel to Europe were stopped. So, as the next best thing, she went to Toronto, and settled down there with the prospect of five pleasant years with a medical qualification at the end.

But she had scarcely arrived when she received a cable from England announcing that she could be granted a passport to go to Oxford on condition that she studied medicine. It was the middle of the war. So many doctors had been killed in France that Britain faced a serious shortage. It had been decided, therefore, to relax the regulations refusing passports to women who were prepared to study medicine.

With trepidation, but knowing that her father would have wished her to go to Oxford, Cicely accepted. Excited and regretful, she said goodbye to all her new friends, and started on the long and hazardous journey to Europe.

Oxford was not what Cicely had dreamed. Because of the war it was an emaciated university both physically and intellectually, and very different from what it had been in Rowland Williams' day. Life was poor and uncomfortable. The students, both men and women, were badly fed and often hungry, though without real hardship. At that time Cicely had not learnt enough about nutrition to know whether or not they suffered from deficiency diseases, but later she suspected that they probably had.

The few male undergraduates had either returned from the front sick or wounded, or else could not join the Army for some definite reason. The town seemed to be full of cadet schools for the Air Force Officer Training Corps. But the women were another matter. Among the forty-one students in Cicely's year there were many to whom, as to Cicely, going up to Oxford was the fulfilment of a lifelong dream. Some had been urged by progressive parents. Others had, from a variety of motives, struggled for their places against prevailing conventions and often against the low educational standards of most girls' schools. There were many young women with similar outlooks and interests. In a short time Cicely had settled down happily with a circle of congenial companions, many of whom remained friends for life.

Apart from the friends she made, her other big experience at Oxford was her introduction to medicine. She was studying only preliminary subjects, biology, chemistry and physics, and later anatomy and physiology, but she already knew that medicine was her vocation.

First-year medical students were not supposed to do clinical work or see patients, but one day she saw a notice announcing that Sir William Osler did a clinic at the Radcliffe Infirmary on Sunday mornings. She sneaked in, and so attended some of the last medical rounds of this great doctor and teacher. She was deeply moved, but only later realised that she had had an amazing introduction to clinical medicine from an outstanding and distinguished teacher. She was particularly impressed by his simple approach to his patients. He was always kindly and an astute observer. He approached patients of different characters in quite different ways. He treated an old lady who obviously enjoyed being demonstrated quite differently from another who was embarrassed by the crowd of students. The only way in which Cicely distinguished herself in these classes was on one occasion when he was demonstrating something not particularly spectacular. She fainted and had to be removed to the ward kitchen, where she was resuscitated with the help of hot tea by the ward sister.

Sir William Osler, on his rounds in Oxford, used to say that priority in medicine was absolute and unvarying. First, service to the patient. Second, teaching of students, whether medical or nursing. Third, research. Cicely never forgot these priorities, and always believed that they should guide any undertaking. She did, however, add a fourth personal priority—the interest and amusement of those who did the work. It always upset her to find doctors, hospitals and even medical schools whose ideas about medical priorities seemed to be different.

Cicely found scientific examinations difficult, and she did badly in her finals. With a poor Third she had to stay at Somerville an extra term to reach the necessary standard in Anatomy and Physiology. But this setback indirectly gave her the distinction of being matriculated as a member of the university on the very first day that women were admitted, early in the autumn term of 1920. She was now living with friends in St Giles and had her own latchkey. Even women of twenty-seven were not allowed latchkeys if they were of undergraduate status.

The presentation of the first degrees ever given to women was a big occasion, and the Sheldonian Theatre was crowded. Even Miss (later Dame) Emily Penrose, the principal of Somerville, had not yet been admitted to the university, so the Somerville women were presented by Professor Gilbert Murray. They wore the new *subfusc* of gowns, black stockings, and specially designed caps, which they all agreed were becoming.

Cicely now had difficulty in finding a place in a hospital for the three years' clinical work she would have to do before qualifying as a doctor. She had understood that her name was on the list at the London Hospital. But by the end of 1919 the hospitals were filling up again with men who had returned from the war. The London Hospital, which had eagerly accepted women students when there was a shortage of men, suddenly decided not to take any more apart from those who had been promised places in writing. Cicely then discovered that her name was not actually entered in the book.

Luckily her youngest brother, who was then at St Thomas's, had a friend at King's College Hospital, which still took women students, and through this small influence she was able to enrol there as a student.

In later life she found it difficult to remember anything that she had not liked at King's. From the moment she arrived she realised that this was what she had lived for. Her later memories were that the whole three years were blissful and the teaching outstanding. The work was arduous, at times as much as twenty hours out of twenty-four. But she found that clinical work was something she was good at, unlike the laboratory work at Oxford which she had never liked. Although most of her contemporaries had begun their hospital work the previous September, she managed after only a few weeks in the hospital to win the Neurology Prize open to First Year students in clinical medicine. It was the first examination that she had ever enjoyed.

In 1923 she passed her Oxford finals after three years at King's College Hospital. She could not have chosen a more difficult time to become a doctor. Most medical students were men who had been in the war. Their careers had been held up while they fought for their country. Naturally everyone wanted to help them and give them jobs. The women, about forty of them at King's during Cicely's time there, were regarded as of comparatively little importance.

Cicely, like any young doctor, would have preferred to start her career with an appointment as House Physician or House Surgeon in her own teaching hospital. But she knew that no women would be selected at King's College Hospital that year, so she didn't even apply. Instead she tried to get a job in another hospital. But here too there were far more young doctors seeking jobs than there were jobs for them to do. There seemed to be no hope of any appointment that would give her good training. Queen Charlotte's, for instance, had no women on the staff. The Hospital for Sick Children in Great Ormond Street, like most other important hospitals, did not accept women in any capacity.

In despair, she looked at the position in private practice. But here, too, few doctors would employ women, and without capital she could not set up in practice on her own.

Desperate, she applied for every job she saw advertised. She sent in between sixty and seventy applications without result. And then at last—partly, she always felt, as the result of a series of mishaps—she was appointed House Physician to the South London Hospital for Women and Children, which was staffed entirely by women.

It turned out to be one of the big breaks of her life. She had to work such long hours that it was three months before she could get out of the hospital for long enough to buy a pair of shoes. The work was constant, day and night, but she revelled in the experience. She worked for several physicians in both the women's and the children's wards, and at the end of her term of office she was reappointed as the House Surgeon of Miss Chadburn, a famous woman pioneer surgeon, which gave her excellent experience in gynaecology.

Miss Chadburn was able, industrious and strict. She expected Cicely to be in touch over every detail, saying, "I wish to keep my finger on the pulse of the hospital." She operated twice a week, starting after lunch and working without a break until after eleven o'clock at night. She reminded Cicely of Queen Victoria, not least because of her height, which was at least eight inches shorter than Cicely's. She had a specially low operating table, and Cicely's back ached so much while she stooped over this table for eight or nine hours at a time that she used to pray for a rope to come from Heaven and support her round the shoulders.

When she finally left the South London Hospital she went to the Queen's Hospital for Children in Hackney,* where a locum doctor was needed. The amount of work was tremendous, the hours of duty arduous, the food and living conditions bad. But Cicely thought that another three weeks of paediatrics would give her what she needed in the way of hospital experience. She then hoped to go into general practice if she could find an assistantship.

But as soon as she started work at this hospital she realised that paediatrics was what she wanted to do for the rest of her life. She stayed for more than a year and was House Physician to Dr Helen Mackay, a distinguished paediatrician whose thinking was in advance of her time. Dr Mackay was already running Child Welfare Clinics on her own, caring for normal children and admitting patients from her clinics into the hospital. This later became accepted practice, but was very unusual then. Working under this system, Cicely soon realised how important it was for the physician to know something about the family. Knowing the mother, being able to advise her, and doing a long-term follow-up were all essential to good child health work. Later, in Africa, this experience led her to organise her work on this basis. The care of the whole child, and everything to do with the child, including the family and especially the mother, was always, to Cicely, the most rational basis on which any sort of child health work should be conducted.

The Queen's Hospital was even busier than the South London. Children queued for admission and many died. Standards of living in the surrounding districts were low. In October the children came to hospital already sewn up in their clothes for the winter. A common pattern of weaning was for the mother to decide that the child was going to be weaned on Sunday, and on Sunday it was taken to Southend-on-Sea and fed on winkles and stout. Cicely had to deal with the consequences on Monday mornings. She learnt much about conditions of life in London at that time. She had to do a great

* Now the Queen Elizabeth Hospital for Children.

deal of her own laboratory work and perform emergency operations. She became skilled at taking out tonsils with a guillotine, and learnt to give anaesthetics for the dentist. When the dentist was tired of pulling out teeth they would swap over, and he would give the anaesthetic while Cicely pulled out the teeth. Later, in Africa, she found that she could remove teeth from a conscious patient without an anaesthetic, and the patient would scarcely realise what had happened.

But it was still a struggle. Doctors, it seemed, were not needed abroad, and women doctors most particularly were not needed. She waited for two years for a post in the Colonial Service, and was told repeatedly that no job was available. But she applied over and over again until eventually she was appointed. As soon as she arrived in Africa she discovered that those who ran the medical services had for years been asking the Colonial Office to send out women doctors, for whom there was a desperate need; yet every time they had asked they were told that none had applied.

Dr Henry O'Hara May, who was a good listener as well as an exuberant talker, barely interrupted Cicely's tale as they strolled in the grounds of the tennis club. When she came to an end he asked her what her impressions were of the Gold Coast.

"I like it tremendously," Cicely replied. "I like everything about it, particularly the Africans. They are marvellous to work with, and I also find the country exciting. I like the way it's all so different wherever you go. I spent three weeks in Kumasi, and I loved the Kwahu scarp and the way it rises hundreds of feet above the forest and runs for hundreds of miles. And the forest itself is so dense and primeval. Going through it I felt I really was descended from the monkey."

"Kumasi, of course, is the Ashanti capital," he said, "and they were once a very war-loving tribe. You can still see the results. But the town has grown big in recent years. Thirty years ago it was an isolated fortress and stood out against a siege. Now it is a great political, cultural and commercial centre. But dealing with the medical services has given me many problems."

"I think you've done it magnificently," Cicely said. "I was told that you were responsible for the new hospital. You seem to have been really inspired when you organised the country's health services on the basis of health clinics for mothers and children and children's and maternity hospitals. I should think it's more developed in the Gold Coast today than in any other British territory."

He smiled and was pleased. She registered this before adding sharply, "You could do with a few more beds, though."

"Oh, you think so, do you?"

"Yes, there are only twelve beds for children and twelve for maternity patients. It's not enough for a growing community of that size. And you need more doctors too. Out-patients is a nightmare. How would you like to see 250 patients in a morning?"

"I'll remember what you say. We can't have our medical officers killed by overwork."

"I don't mind overwork," she slashed back, "but it's not fair on the patients. How can they get proper treatment under those conditions?"

"You are quite right, my dear," he said soothingly. "I'll see what can be done. And now let's go and have a drink in the club house."

The bar of the tennis club was crowded, and as they entered there were cries of "Well done, Henry", "Well played, Henry!". O'Hara May passed a few joking comments, bought two iced lagers and retreated with Cicely.

"Ah," he said, sinking into a comfortable chair and signalling to the waiter to move the table nearer. "Just the thing after tennis."

"Or after a long, hot clinic," she reminded him.

"I forgot you were working this afternoon. How are you enjoying the work in Christiansborg?"

"Very much. It's not so hectic as in Kumasi."

"Can you diagnose the diseases? Apart from diphtheria, of course. We all know your competence in that."

She laughed. "I can usually spot something straightforward like T.B., malaria or yaws. But one sees so many diseases that are different from anything one was taught. There is one condition in particular that worries me."

She told him about the twins and their peeling skins and fading reddish hair.

"I've seen children like that, of course," he said, "but I never thought of it as a specific disease. So many diseases out here are unlike anything described. It's difficult to sort them out."

"Especially in children. Children's diseases aren't really on the map yet." Her face had become intense.

He smiled. "That's something for you to do. It'll keep you out of mischief."

"When I've been here a little longer and learnt some languages."

"What are you going to do about that? You must pass an exam in an African language before you can be confirmed in your appointment."

"I've decided to learn Twi. I gather that it's the Ashanti language and is spoken over much of the country."

"A sensible choice. I chose Ga myself and it was two years between I even knew the difference between Yes and No. Are you going to have lessons?"

"I've started already with the wife of a missionary who lives in Christiansborg. What's more . . ." Her face betrayed a little boasting smile, "I already know the word for 'worms' in six African languages."

He was delighted. "That's *exactly* the right approach." He slapped his thigh and gulped cold lager. "You've only got to learn as many words for 'syphilis' and you really will be a tropical doctor."

CHAPTER II

SHE WAS TIRED when she got back to her bungalow, a small but adequate concrete hut in an area specially demarcated for Europeans. Government employees had to live in these areas because of the danger of yellow fever. This was before the days of inoculations, and during an epidemic most of the Europeans who got the disease died. Other deadly diseases such as blackwater fever were also far from uncommon.

Bare earth stretched round the house, compulsorily. Even a tin or bottle hidden in the grass might encourage mosquitoes to breed and infect people with malaria or yellow fever.

She pushed open the door which led straight into the sparsely furnished main room. The manservant had left it tidy and reasonably clean. Cicely would have preferred a woman, but this was not permitted. Because of the ever present danger of infection, the menservants had to leave their wives and children in the African residential areas.

In the middle of the room stood a large wooden table with each of its feet in a tin of water to stop the ants. But tins brought their own dangers, and could easily become breeding grounds for dangerous mosquito larvae. The water had to be changed frequently and the regulations were strict and ruthlessly enforced. There were frequent public health inspections. Even medical officers were not exempt, and Cicely had already been fined for having larvae in a flower vase.

She was up early next morning ready to drive to the clinic soon after seven o'clock in the small Morris that she had bought fifth-hand from her predecessor. It coughed and spluttered, and she wondered whether there could be sand in the carburettor. Suddenly the engine roared and the pipe seemed to have cleared itself. Relieved and jubilant, she raced along the sandy road that led to the clinic.

It was "Yaws morning". This would mean that there would be about 150 infected children to inject with bismuth salicylate. There would be much yelling, and it would be necessary to work hard to persuade the mothers to bring their children for further treatment. The cure was not rapid or spectacular, but most of the cases did well, provided they came regularly for six injections.

Already across the courtyard stretched a long line of waiting patients, mostly mothers and children. A few children were alone or accompanied by brothers and sisters. Many had visible signs of the disease. Some of the smaller children had sores on their faces or buttocks, showing that they had probably caught the disease while being carried on their infected mothers' backs. Some limped because of yaws on the feet. A few had extensive destruction of bone. Cicely never got used to seeing nose and mouth as one gaping hole. These cases upset her most of all because she knew that they were preventable.

Only the day before she had been telling the African nurses how yaws could be largely prevented by cleanliness, saying, "Look, I am handling children with yaws all day long, but I wash my hands and I don't get yaws." But now she found the nurses busy polishing the clinic. She called to one who was attacking a metal dish with a bottle of Bluebell, and said laughingly, "Nurse, that's not really the sort of cleaning I meant when we talked about preventing yaws. Needles of bismuth is what these patients need."

The nurse looked up and grinned. "No, Missee Dokiter, this not yaws treatment. Lady Governor, she come today. Yaws day. She come in fine big car. She fine lady need everything shiny."

Then Cicely remembered. The health services in Ghana were greatly assisted by voluntary workers. One of the voluntary workers who came to help on yaws days was Lady Slater, the Governor's wife. Cicely had not yet met her because the Governor and his wife had been away on leave.

"Right, nurse, let's start," said Cicely, peering into the electric steriliser. It was bubbling quietly in the corner, filled with syringes.

She did about fifty injections on her own. The nurse was fully occupied at the steriliser. This meant that Cicely had to fill each syringe herself before giving the injection. A voluntary worker to fill the syringes would double the speed of work.

An enormous black Rolls Royce slid into the compound. Cicely washed her hands, and went to meet her distinguished helper. Lady Slater was good-looking and majestic, but also down-to-earth. She greeted Cicely, and asked whether she was settling into her bungalow.

"What are you doing about curtains?"

"I've brought some stuff with me and I'm going to make them myself."

"How energetic of you. Have you a sewing machine?"

"No. but it won't take too long to run them up by hand."

"You are obviously clever with needles," smiled Lady Slater, filling the first syringe.

There were still about fifty injections to do when the main fuse blew. Cicely managed to mend it, but it instantly blew again. There was enough light from the sun to see what she was doing, but there was no longer any means of sterilising the syringes.

"Do you think we can get an electrician along quickly?" asked Cicely anxiously. She was afraid that if the patients had to wait too long they would go away without the treatment that she felt they needed so badly.

"Not a hope," said Lady Slater. "I've been in this country long enough to know that there won't be any chance of getting it done till tomorrow. But we keep a big primus stove at Government House for emergencies. I could go and get it."

When she had gone, Cicely and the nurse walked down the long line of patients trying to make them understand what had happened and, still more important, that if only they would wait a while they would get their important treatment. This was not easy, because among those fifty patients some seven or eight or even more languages were spoken. Although the nurse could manage three or four languages, there were still a few patients who did not understand. One of these was a tall striking woman with a droopy baby. Cicely drew her from the queue. She didn't like the look of the baby.

The nurse managed to find a man who spoke both the woman's language and one that the nurse could understand. Cicely started to conduct the interview through these two interpreters. It seemed to her that the conversation went something like this:

Cicely to nurse-interpreter: "Ask her how long the baby has been sick.'

Nurse to second interpreter: "Bongo, Bonga, Bonga, Wong."

Second interpreter to mother: "Wula, Wula, Wula, Wa."

A long argument followed between the second interpreter and the mother. Then the nurse intervened, and it all came back again. Finally the nurse-interpreter folded her hands in her lap and said, "Please, doctor, she says 'yes'."

Cicely gave up trying to take the history, put the baby on a couch and began to examine him. His heart was failing but she couldn't find out why.

"He must go to hospital immediately," she said. "Now. This afternoon. Somehow you've got to get her to understand. The baby will die if he doesn't go."

She wondered again, as she did so often, why so many children were dying of diseases that neither she nor anyone else could diagnose.

The next patient was a young girl. Like most Africans she did not know her age accurately, but Cicely guessed that she was about eighteen. She was pregnant and, like many others, had arrived with her mother, father, husband, grandparents and other relatives too. After examining her Cicely explained that she would have to have a Caesarean operation. This was apparently unknown in Christiansborg. While Cicely was trying to explain the situation to the girl and to her husband, parents, grandparents and other relatives, rumours buzzed up and down the line of waiting patients and the nurse reported that the whole idea was causing a sensation in the crowd. Eventually, after much argument, Cicely succeeded in persuading the girl to go to the maternity hospital in Accra. A few weeks later she came back with a healthy baby. This caused even more of a sensation. She described what she had been through, how she had known nothing about it and had suffered no pain, and how she had woken up and found a cut down her belly and a fine baby beside her. For months afterwards women in labour would scream, saying, "Cut me open, don't let me have a baby this way. Let me have it through my belly."

Eventually Lady Slater returned, bringing with her not only a primus stove, paraffin and saucepan, but also the sewing machine for Cicely's curtains.

"You must come to our party," she said at the end of the day. "We're going to have a big one at Christmas."

It was a good party, too, held in the magnificent fortress of Christiansborg castle. Sir Alfred and Lady Slater invited all the unattached men and women who were considered suitable. The doctors went dressed as pirates. Cicely was persuaded to dance the apache dance again, and ended the evening being piloted round the ballroom on the handlebars of somebody's bicycle. Next day she received a letter from one of her aunts in England commiserating with her for spending Christmas so far from home. The letter said, "I wonder whether you are having a lonely Christmas dinner or whether you are sharing it with some other lonely soul?"

"I want to talk to you seriously, Cicely," said Dr O'Hara May.

They had dined in the European Club, talking light-heartedly of many things and discovering more interests in common. Now they were drinking liqueurs in the half-light of the verandah. Cicely studied his face and waited. Eventually he said, "How's the work going?"

"Fine on the whole." She shrugged her shoulders slightly. "At least, I seem to get through a lot."

"You sound as though you doubt its worth."

"No. But I think we probably give ourselves a good deal of extra trouble."

"How do you mean?"

"In a way we're becoming too popular. Take vaccination, for instance. I think it's important that all the children should be vaccinated, so I buy huge tins of sweets. Every child gets a sweet with the injection, and now they seem to come just for the sweet. I suspect that I am vaccinating a large proportion of the child population of Christiansborg at weekly intervals."

He laughed. "Yes, I know that tends to happen. It's difficult to avoid."

"If only we could keep records," said Cicely. "In England patients have cards and we notice if they come too often."

"I don't see how we could have records here," O'Hara May said. "At least, not for inoculations and so on. For one thing, Africans don't have permanent names and addresses. Also we haven't the staff. We are almost bound to be either ignored or else too popular. I prefer the latter."

"Popularity isn't the end of the world," said Cicely, "but it's a waste of time when there's so much to be done."

"That's one of the things I want to talk to you about," he said. "In a way we've got things organised down here on the Coast. The need is greater up country. Except for a few centres such as Kumasi, we're doing very little and only reaching a small fraction of the Africans."

"I thought we were supposed to be so advanced in the Gold Coast," she said mockingly. "And that you were the inspiration and source of it all."

He smiled sadly and said, "It's kind of you to say so, Cicely. We may be advanced in comparison with some other colonies, but not by any real standards. It's true that we've had a lot of money to spend on the medical services—getting on for a quarter of a million a year. And building the hospital at Korle Bu took another quarter of a million or more. But even so the services are pitifully inadequate. The child mortality is fantastically high."

"Shouldn't we be training more Africans?" she asked.

"Yes. The present situation is disgraceful. There's woefully little higher education available for Africans. Of course, there's Achimota College. That provides co-education of a kind for

Africans from kindergarten to university, and it's good in its way. Dr Fraser, the principal, is first-rate. But in a way the very success of Achimota College makes the whole situation worse. The college is expensive and so, of course, the Government is reluctant to spend money elsewhere as well. The result is that, in the whole country, we have about two African doctors and no African engineers, scientists or architects at all."

"There seem to be plenty of African lawyers," said Cicely. "I'm always hearing of Africans being promoted to posts as judges, magistrates and so on."

"That's about the only thing they do go in for," he said. "God knows why. I don't know whether it's just a symptom of their interest in litigation or whether it's an active Government policy to turn them into lawyers and nothing else. Of course, it's very much Lord Lugard's idea that Africans should learn self-government by means of their own self-appointed methods of government through their own chiefs, and I suppose we're trying to support this by training them in law. But it will be disastrous if it's not supported by Africans with the right professional training in other fields."

"What have I to do with all this?" asked Cicely. He obviously had something up his sleeve.

"Well, my dear, of all the medical officers I have ever had out here, you are the only one who has really understood what I am trying to do and why. So I'm sending you to Koforidua to organise the maternal and child health services. At the moment, in spite of all our talk, the women and children there are getting practically no medical care at all. Now how do you feel about that?"

"Oh, marvellous," said Cicely, without hesitation. "I'd love to do it if you think I can."

"I'm sure you can."

"What's it like there? Koforidua is the cocoa town, isn't it?"

"That's right. It's only about fifty miles away and has about 10,000 inhabitants. Half the world's cocoa comes from the Gold Coast and about half of that from Koforidua. It's rich, and very

African. Europeans aren't allowed to own land, so big firms like Cadbury and United Africa have to buy their cocoa at market prices. All the money, and there's plenty of it, goes back to the Africans. But the medical services are terrible. The children are dying like flies."

The verandah was quiet. The dim ceiling light was reflected in Cicely's liqueur glass and threw back a tiny beam across the table.

"I shall miss Accra," she said. "But I'm pleased you're sending me away. It may sound silly, but I already feel I know what to do."

Koforidua was just as O'Hara May had said. There was a hospital with a doctor in charge, but nearly all the patients were men. The medical services did not seem to concern themselves with women and children, though these constituted three-quarters of the population.

She was given a new bungalow on the edge of the forest, in the area allotted to Europeans, and also one room in the office of the Medical Officer of Health, where she was told to start maternal and child health work, though without hospital beds.

The Medical Officer of Health was an elderly Irishman with a good knowledge of Africa and a liking for efficiency and golf. This meant that, whatever else was done or left undone, the cellar was always stocked, the sanitary services were well run and the grass on the golf course was cut, rolled and swept. While she was in Koforidua Cicely became quite a competent player. But on at least one occasion she stayed indoors. This was during a plague of flying ants, and few people left their houses, except on the most essential business. The M.O.H. went out swathed in scarves with trousers tucked into top boots instead of the usual shirt and shorts, and attended by three small boys, one to carry his clubs, one to watch the ball and a third armed with a small branch. As he stood to address the ball, he was lightly switched all over with the branch and so was the ball. Then came a brief pause, and swoosh went the ball.

Cicely wondered how he felt about giving her a room in his office, and she was anxious to make friends with him, hoping to enlist his co-operation. The attitude of the Medical Officer of Health could make all the difference between success and failure. She apologised for inconveniencing him and tried to draw him out.

"So you've come to do maternal and child care work?" he said benevolently, but with a hint of scepticism in his voice.

"Yes," said Cicely hesitantly, wondering what he would say next. There was a pause and he stared at her carefully, before saying sharply:

"Well, you'd better get on and do it."

He seemed about to stump out of the room. Cicely spoke quickly to detain him.

"But I can't start just like that. How will the patients know? We must go out into the town and into the surrounding villages and talk to the people and persuade the women to bring their children."

"That won't be necessary," said the M.O.H. "I know these people. You won't need any propaganda. They'll come to you from far and wide. But whether or not you'll do them any good is another matter."

"How do you mean?" she asked earnestly, and saw instantly that it was the wrong thing to say.

"What do I mean?" he repeated, testily. "What I mean is that you people come out here to reform the place when you don't know the first thing about it. All you do is make a mess of things and stir up trouble."

"But mothers and babies . . ." Cicely started to defend herself.

"Mothers and babies twaddle," he said. "Whatever will it be next? These people have too many babies anyway. Why do you want to encourage them to have more? You'd be better employed having babies of your own, my girl."

He was angry now, and glowering.

"Here, look at that." With a dramatic gesture of crushing her he flung her a newspaper.

Bewildered, Cicely looked at it. It was Koforidua's weekly newspaper in English. The doctor's big forefinger pointed to the correspondence column. Cicely read, "To the Editor. Dear Sir,

Is it correct for a Medical Officer to Health to treat us with insults? At a certain village a discussion was held, at the end of which the M.O.H. departed saying, 'You seem to expect the Government to come and wipe your bloody backsides for you.' (Signed) Indignant."

Cicely was aware that the M.O.H. was watching her, pleased to embarrass and shock her. She started to laugh, at first in a giggle and then long and loud.

"What's so funny?" he asked, surprised and a little indignant.

"I think it's very funny," Cicely said, still laughing.

"All right," he said, belligerently. "If you think it's so funny, what do you think I should do about it?"

"I suggest that you persuade the village to adopt as its motto 'Our backs are bloody but unbowed'!"

The M.O.H. started to laugh too, and slapped her on the back. Then he fetched a second whisky glass and said they must celebrate, and in a few minutes she knew that she had made another friend.

He told her that there were only five European women in Koforidua, and she was the first unmarried lady ever to be posted there. As a result the many bachelors had organised a "Bachelors' Preservation Association".

"Very well," said Cicely. "Here and now I form a Spinsters' Protection Society of which I shall be president, secretary, treasurer and members, all in one."

"I suspect," said the M.O.H., refilling his whisky glass while Cicely hastily covered hers with her hand, "that the Bachelors' Preservation Association will soon invite the Spinsters' Protection Society to join them lock, stock and barrel."

And so it turned out.

The supply of patients was also as the M.O.H. foretold. On the first morning Cicely left for her office wondering how easy it would be to persuade the women to come to the clinic and how long it would take for the news to spread. In spite of what the M.O.H. had said she still had a feeling that no one would want to come and see her or to bring their children.

To her astonishment at least thirty patients were waiting outside the door.

"See," said the M.O.H. triumphantly.

Next day there were more than fifty patients waiting, and some of them had come long distances.

"The people are great travellers," said the old doctor. "They are always going from the town to the villages and from the villages to their farms, and they all know what's going on in the other parts of the country. The people here have heard about the children's clinics in Accra and Kumasi. As soon as they heard there was a doctor coming to Koforidua who was particularly interested in children, nothing kept them back."

Next day there were even more patients waiting, and Cicely began to feel confident that her maternal and child care work was going to succeed.

But on the fourth day she saw a very ill child with spots, and was told that there were more sick children with spots on the edge of the town. Next day there were still more sick children with spots from other parts of the town, and from the countryside too. On the same day, the M.O.H. went sick. Cicely realised that she was virtually in sole charge of an extensive epidemic of smallpox.

This would be a gruelling test of all that she had been taught and trained to do. She had only been in Africa a few months, and knew little of African conditions and ways of life. But smallpox was one of the most infectious and fatal diseases in the world.

"The first essential," she announced, "is to vaccinate as many people as possible, particularly those who have been in contact with cases of the disease and those who wish to travel from one area to another."

With some difficulty road blocks were set up on all the roads round Koforidua. Anyone who wished to travel had to have a pass, and nobody could get one who had not been recently vaccinated. Then the town and villages had to be combed in the search for new cases. Once mass vaccination was organised patients came in hundreds. But the number of cases of smallpox increased every day. Nursing them became a problem, which was overcome by getting patients who had recovered to nurse new cases. Cicely was delighted to see how quickly they learnt to wash the other patients, give them fluids, keep them warm and generally look after them. These emergency village hospitals multiplied and practised medicine at its most primitive level.

She was pleased, too, to find that vaccination was so popular among the people. On one occasion she received a message from the chief of Koforidua himself saying that he wanted the "woman doctor" to come and vaccinate the women of his household. She was told that there might be fifty or sixty of them with their children. But before she was allowed to go home she had vaccinated over 300 people. As soon as she had done one batch, a request came that this was an uncle of the chief or his nephew, and he too had a family. It struck her that there was prestige attached to the fact of being vaccinated by a white woman.

But the popularity of vaccination was not universal. A number of people, particularly women, would come and display big keloid scars on their arms, three of them together imitating smallpox vaccination. They had got themselves scarified and had then rubbed in some irritating substance, probably the skin of the cashew nut, in order to produce the keloid.

At last the epidemic had passed its peak, though it was by no means yet controlled. Dr O'Hara May came up from Accra. Cicely was so involved with her work that she could scarcely greet him.

"I'm just going out to visit a suspect village," she said. "I daren't omit it yet, even for a day."

"I'll come with you," he said, though he was tired from his journey from the capital. "It intrigues me to know how you find all these cases so quickly. You seem to be diagnosing them almost before they get ill."

"It's simple," she said, smiling. In spite of her compulsion not to pause in her work, she was delighted to see him. "Of course, the villagers often try to conceal smallpox because they don't want their movements to be restricted. But they put white rags on the trees and hedges to keep away the evil spirits. You just drive round in the evenings, and wherever you see white rags you know that they've got smallpox. The health inspectors are very good at observing and reporting."

Later that evening, the tour over, they sat quietly together. Henry O'Hara May said, "Cicely, you're doing a good job of work up here."

She muttered, "It's only just beginning." But she was pleased. "It's funny," she said. "Through all these difficulties and worries there is one thought that keeps recurring in my mind, though it's quite unrealistic."

"Yes?" he said, encouragingly.

"I wish my father could see me now," she said. "He always wanted me to become a woman doctor, but I don't believe he thought I would achieve it."

Once the smallpox epidemic was under control Cicely again devoted her attention to starting the clinic in the M.O.H.'s office. A new clinic was being built, but would not be ready for some months.

Again the number of patients increased rapidly. As soon as the doors were opened there were surging masses of stalwart mammies, African women carrying children, dragging children, pushing children. Sometimes Cicely was afraid the children would be crushed to death. Soon she had to have police to keep the crowds at bay. It was embarrassing to be so popular. Women and children travelled long distances to see her, and anybody coming into the market would bring their children to the clinic.

Success filled her with pride and hope and greatly increased her confidence. She began to feel that most of what she had been told was wrong and most of what she felt was right. The women of Ghana were primitive and ignorant, but they were not apathetic or stupid. Many were highly intelligent and full of initiative and vigour. They wanted the best for their children, and they recognised it when they saw it.

But the work itself became nightmarish. One room served for waiting, consulting, examination, treatment, sterilising and dispensing. Cicely had no dispenser or nurse to help her, and was entirely on her own except for a young African girl who could speak three or four of the local languages and enough English to make do. Between them they coped with over a hundred patients a day. Most of the children who came were sick, and Cicely had to do all the treatments herself. Most common were cases of scabies, which she had to treat on the spot and show the mothers how to do the treatment. She had to dress the many ulcers, give all the injections for yaws and malaria, and do all the microscope work, looking for dysentery and worms. She also had to give out all the medicine. One day, working entirely on her own, she saw more than 160 patients. There was so much work that there was no time to organise it properly. Moreover, she became so obsessed with the importance of what she was doing that she was unable to appreciate the importance of tailoring the work to suit her facilities. The needs of the African women and their children and the realisation that she had found an effective way to help them possessed her beyond all proportions.

She began to sleep badly. She would find herself sitting up in bed at night as though her bedroom door was being battered down by mothers coming in all night long. She would call out, "You can't come in now. You must wait until the morning." But still the long queues seemed to hammer the door.

In trying to sort out her thoughts she began at weekends to make a garden outside her bungalow. But one of the difficulties was the enormous number of midges in this area just outside the forest. As soon as she went into the garden she was bitten atrociously. She developed a rash all over and her temperature rose. She went to see the doctor in charge at the hospital, who said, "Oh, that's just a bit of prickly heat." She was certain that it was not prickly heat. The doctor had not noticed that she had a fever, and she felt too miserable to point it out to him. She went to work. It so happened that her car had gone to the garage for repairs. A friend drove her to the clinic, but when it was time to go home at midday no one remembered to pick her up. Again she was too miserable to complain, and she walked home two miles. When she arrived home she found that her temperature was over 103°, but, overcome by the thought of the queue of patients waiting for the afternoon clinic, she walked back again after lunch and finished the day's work with the rash getting worse all the time. During the long, hot clinic she controlled the fever and, to some extent, the symptoms by taking aspirin at frequent intervals.

Next day she was no better, but again she went to work. She continued to work throughout her illness with a proud and stubborn toughness that was a growing feature of her character. Bowing to illness betrayed a weakness that she was reluctant to admit. In later years she was to experience the most extreme conditions that the human body can stand, and this practised toughness became important in survival.

Two weeks later the wife of the hospital doctor developed the same illness. Her husband put her to bed and sent for a special nurse to come up from Accra to look after her. Cicely, working on in the clinic, had feelings of resentful triumph.

After the fever subsided she was left with a painful arthritis. The joints of her fingers were affected, and the worst place of all was the left side of her jaw. Eating was painful, and she was always being caught out because she had discovered automatically that when you are examining a child whose language you do not speak, and you want him to open his mouth, you instinctively open your own to show him what you mean.

Twice again she had these attacks of fever with a rash, but each one was less serious. She came to the conclusion that the illness was an allergic reaction to the bites of the midges, to which one gradually developed immunity. She noticed that no Africans seemed to get the disease. After her third attack the midges had no effect. She could take her trowel and scrape them from her arms and not feel their bites.

At the end of her illness Dr O'Hara May came up from Accra and was shocked by what he found. He spoke to her most seriously.

"Cicely, my dear, however strongly you feel about it, you can't take on the whole of Africa. You'll only kill yourself and then no one will benefit. It would be far better to do less work and organise it more sensibly."

She admitted that she had been overdoing things.

"I suppose," she said ruefully, "that one of the things that has saved my life has been the fact that there was no lighting in the office. I've been starting the clinic soon after dawn, but I had to close it at dusk. Otherwise I should probably have gone on all night. But all the same, you know," and her face lit up with enthusiasm, "we must extend this work more and more. It's terribly important. By these methods we can save many thousands of lives and, perhaps even more important, we can prevent ill health before it ever occurs. Why don't we get on and do it?"

"It sounds simple," said O'Hara May. "But two big essentials, as you've already found out to your cost, are facilities and organisation, and that's what I want to talk to you about rather than about the big problem of the health of Africa. Now, first of all, containers for medicines. Would it help if every patient brought with her a bottle and a tin?"

Thus Cicely's feet came once more to earth and she began to organise the clinic. The patients soon learned to help in bringing their own equipment, usually a rinsed gin bottle and a cigarette tin. These were filled from bottles and jars of stock mixture from the hospital. She began to study the faces of the patients, and realised that many came out of idleness and inquisitiveness. Others came repeatedly, apparently believing that the more often you visited the doctor and the more medicine you drank, the quicker you would get well. "We have broken the bottle," they would say. "You must give us another one." Large numbers of women came to the antenatal clinic whether they were pregnant or not. Many of those who were pregnant tried to come every day. Cicely told them firmly, "You mustn't come here for another month unless there is really something wrong with you." She started to issue cards for each patient with the name written on it with a serial number, and on the back she wrote the dates on which they attended. The notes were brief but specific, and enabled her to keep some control of what was happening. She tried to remember the faces of the women who came saying that they had lost their cards.

By the time the new buildings were opened by the Provincial Commissioner in an impressive ceremony Cicely felt that she had mastered the work. She now had a consulting room, examination room, treatment room and a dispensary, all with verandahs where patients could wait, and with proper sanitary facilities. She also had a nurse, a midwife and a dispenser, and reckoned that with this team she could see up to 250 patients a day. The midwife was also called Williams. She came from Sierra Leone, and had been trained in England. Cicely found her a great asset to the work in Koforidua. Although she could not speak the local languages well, her English was good, and being a slight foreigner in the place she acted as a sort of intermediary for Cicely.

O'Hara May came up from Accra for the celebrations and was delighted at the change. He hugged her affectionately.

"This is a triumph for you, Cicely. How do you feel?"

"Wonderful," she said, radiant. "I feel pleased and triumphant. But I also have the feeling that it's only a small and essential beginning to something much bigger and more important."

"Interesting. Have you ever felt like this before?"

"I think so." She was silent for a moment, trying to identify the memory precisely. "I think I felt almost exactly as I feel tonight when I first arrived in Oxford."

Now that the clinic buildings were finished, her work became even more popular. In spite of the improved facilities the queues of patients began to grow again, and so did the numbers of those who abused the service. Visiting the white lady doctor had become a fashionable occupation for African ladies, and there was no way to stop them from coming to the clinic over and over again. Her system of issuing cards which would keep some check on their visits was difficult to work—for a patient who wished to take advantage could conveniently lose her card and had to be given another. It was also impossible to keep an alphabetical index. Ten boys called Kofi might attend on the same morning, and in any case the Africans changed their names frequently and also those of their children.

The amount of work was sometimes almost intolerable, but Cicely continued to organise her thoughts. What she saw was quite different from what she had learnt at the London School of Tropical Medicine. There the pattern of disease had been taught systematically, classified neatly as though diseases have some life of their own apart from the people in whom they occur. She could often recognise these as vague background patterns to what she actually saw in the clinic.

She was particularly worried about the condition which she had already noticed in Accra; it was common, and often fatal, and was not described in the textbooks. Many children were brought to her with swollen bellies and legs, and sometimes with their skin peeling; nearly all were miserable. They might have had beri-beri due to deficiency of vitamin B1—but when she gave them this vitamin they did not improve. She had no idea what the condition was, and she began to study it. The children were often of a lighter colour than their parents. Sometimes there was a reddish tinge to their hair, and some had a peculiar rash. In the late stages the skin became thick and black and peeled off easily, and soon after this the children usually died.

But she made little progress in her research. She had no hospital beds or laboratory, so it was impossible to study the patients continuously or do the necessary scientific investigations.

She was lying in bed one night, awake and anxious about the future of her clinic. O'Hara May was due to visit next day, and she was thinking of all the things she hoped to say to him.

She also felt uneasy for a more sinister reason. Some months before she had heard rumours of human sacrifice, but she had taken little notice at the time. Now something had happened which brought it to her mind. The previous day an important local chief had died. Cicely's servants were both Nigerian, and they came to her, terrified, and said that they could not possibly go shopping.

"Why are you frightened?"

"The king of England has given permission for ten foreigners to be used as human sacrifices for the chief's funeral. We may be chosen because we are from Nigeria!"

"Nonsense! Whoever told you that is telling lies. The English king would never give such permission." Cicely was definite in her reassurances, but she was left with unpleasant feelings.

It was about three o'clock in the morning and suddenly she heard shouting. Someone was coming up the hill towards her bungalow. Then there was more shouting. She suppressed her fear and decided that it might be a parent whose child had died and who needed a death certificate so that the body could be buried at once. This happened occasionally because it was the custom to bury the body quickly.

Someone knocked. She decided not to answer, but then heard the familiar voice of her neighbour, George Warner, a policeman.

"Dr Williams, can you come quickly? There's been an accident."

Lying on the settee in the policeman's bungalow was his servant, bleeding heavily from half a hand. Cicely could see that his thumb and two first fingers had been cut off with a sharp instrument.

"I didn't hear a thing," said Warner. "His groaning woke me."

Together they unravelled the story. The boy said that he had been woken in the night and found two Ashanti men in his room, and when he heard the noise he shouted to the other boy, "Kwami, but it no be Kwami", and then he called, "Kojo, but it no be Kojo." Then the Ashanti men came in, attacked him with a machete, and left him with only two fingers on his left hand.

Cicely was giving the boy first aid and preparing to take him to hospital, when there was more shouting. Lights flashed, and in burst some colleagues of Warner's in the police force.

The true story gradually emerged and was very different. The boy had gone to a gin shop in Koforidua, attacked the shopkeeper and tried to steal bottles of gin. The shopkeeper had defended himself with a machete and had cut off the boy's fingers. The police had followed the stream of blood all the way from the gin shop nearly a mile away, up the valley, over the bridge and along the road to George Warner's house.

Cicely was astonished at the presence of mind with which the boy had invented the story, including the details about Kwami and Kojo, while walking up the hill with half his hand lopped off.

With difficulty, she switched her mind back to the problem of card index systems in the clinic.

"What do you think should be done about it?" asked Dr O'Hara May. They were sitting comfortably on the verandah of Cicely's bungalow discussing the success and problems of the new clinic.

She said, "I think I know what the solution is, but I don't think you'll like it."

"Let's have it."

"I think we ought to make the patients pay a fee. I know it's Government policy to provide free out-patient treatment for Africans in all hospitals, and on the whole I think that's a good principle. But as things are at the moment I think we'd give better treatment to more patients if we did charge."

"It's a novel idea," he said thoughtfully. "But not really revolutionary. Tell me how you're thinking of organising it."

Without the half-expected rebuff, she warmed to the theme.

"I think the most important thing is to charge for cards. We started issuing them some time ago to keep some check on what's going on and to prevent the patients from visiting us over and over again just for the pleasure of seeing us. But as long as the cards are free, the patients can keep them or lose them according to convenience. I believe this is one of the reasons why we're so overcrowded. If they had to pay, say, a shilling for a new card, and possibly sixpence for each subsequent attendance, I think they would have more respect for the treatment."

"What about the really poor people?"

"There's not much real poverty in this part of Africa. Many people are so prosperous that they employ others to do their work and live a life of leisure. It's the richer women who tend to be the most nuisance because they haven't enough to do and coming to the clinic helps to fill in time. But there are a few genuine hard cases, and we could let them come free. I also think we needn't charge patients who really need to attend frequently. Although I don't like the principle of making patients pay, I think that a system like this would improve our standard of treatment."

"All right," said O'Hara May. "You seem to know what you are talking about. You go ahead and do what you bloody well like."

Then she told him about the mysterious disease.

"We talked of this before," he said.

"I first noticed it in Christiansborg. But the more I study it, the more convinced I am that we're on to something important, certainly for the Gold Coast, and perhaps for other parts of the world too."

She was right. Kwashiorkor, as the disease was later called, turned out to be one of the world's biggest problems.

Cicely later identified it and found the cure, but even today it kills more children in the world than any other disease.

"But what can I do?" she went on. "We have no laboratories or hospital beds."

"Do you think it's an infection?"

"I think that it's something more generally environmental. Nutritional, perhaps."

"You mean a vitamin deficiency?"

"Not really. I've tried all the vitamins and none of them makes any difference. I think our whole thought is wrong."

"How do you propose to find out more?"

"Well, I can't, can I?" She flung out her hands despairingly. "Without a laboratory and without hospital beds I can do nothing."

The pitch of her voice had risen across the quiet, bare garden, now filled, thanks to Cicely's work, with petunias, nasturtiums and zinnias. O'Hara May sat quietly and drew on his pipe.

"I wasn't going to tell you this, Cicely, but I believe you're on to something important. Soon another job will be vacant in Accra, and I want you to have it. You'll be in charge of the Children's Hospital and have research facilities in the laboratories at Korle Bu. Would you like that?"

"Oh, very much," she gasped.

"You should be able to build up a first-class children's unit there."

"When can I start?"

"First of all I want you to have a really good holiday. You've worked continuously ever since you came out here. I think you need a rest and a change."

"Nonsense. I only need a brief pause. Actually I am due a couple of weeks' local leave, and I've been invited to stay with the Goslings at Aburi, and go with them for a few days by the sea at Prampram."

Her holiday was nearly disastrous. She enjoyed swimming in the sea so much that she failed to notice the currents. She was pulled out half drowned by a passing fisherman. After that she felt so full of health and energy that for several days she forgot to take the quinine which everyone was supposed to take every night. The result was a severe attack of malaria, verging on blackwater fever, a particularly dangerous form of the disease. After this she was ordered to go on leave at once, and she went home to Jamaica for two months.

CHAPTER III

She returned to Accra to take charge of the Princess Marie Louise Hospital for Children, and promptly had her first serious disagreement with her friend and chief, Dr Henry O'Hara May. It concerned dying children.

Many of the children under her care were dying. And she knew that the mysterious disease was responsible for many of these deaths. But it was one thing to recognise the disease. It was another to understand it and find its cause.

It was impossible to investigate the cause of death because few children actually died in the hospital. When a mother saw that her child was dying she would drag it out of bed, tie it on to her back and hurry home by bus or lorry. Cicely suffered deeply when the children died. She also knew that until she could do post-mortems she had no hope of discovering the cause of the disease or its cure.

She went to see O'Hara May in his office to suggest that some means be found for stopping this practice. She found him adamant and unusually lacking in sympathy.

"Cicely, I know how much you care about this. But you can't go against the wishes of the people. Post-mortems would be directly against not only their customs, but also their religion."

"How do you know?" asked Cicely bitterly.

"Well, I suppose I can't actually prove it. One never can prove what one knows about African life and ways. But I am sure that according to the customs and religion of these people anyone who is dying must be taken home and buried there before sunset. They've always done this, and there's been no change in the custom in all the years I've been out here. I don't think you could change it now, and I think it would be unwise to try to do so. You've built up a tremendous amount of good-will among African women since you came here. They're beginning to know you and trust you, and you're in an excellent position to do really first-class health work. Don't throw it all away by antagonising them. You'd lose more than you'd gain."

She was unconvinced. When her feelings were roused she could be stubborn and determined.

She was beginning to speak several African languages. She decided to try to talk to the mothers, and learn more of how they felt.

One of the difficulties was the tradition of silence among Ghanaian people concerning certain words. For instance, it was regarded as bad luck to utter aloud the word for "whooping-cough", so when a child had whooping-cough the mother would tie a key round its neck and this would tell the doctor that it had whooping-cough and also that the word must not be mentioned. It was clear that there were also customs of silence concerning the mystery disease. Any attempt to discuss it with the mothers or to question them was met with a curious emotional response. Cicely found it difficult to analyse, but it seemed to be chiefly a mixture of embarrassment, excitement and fear. The response of the African nurses was also peculiar. Cicely felt sure that they had thoughts and feelings on the subject, but any attempt to elicit them produced a reaction that was only slightly more sophisticated than that of the patients.

She was beginning to understand some of the mysterious forms of communication that were so much more developed in Africans than in Europeans. She felt that she could communicate with the women in their own medium. She had also realised that as she got to know people better they were more likely to mention unmentionable words.

Every night, sometimes on her way home from a dinner party, she returned to the hospital to do a round of the wards. She had done this since her arrival in Accra, but now she began to include conversation with mothers in her regular round. She felt sure that if only she persevered long enough she would obtain from them some of the information she needed.

It was the custom for mothers to go into hospital with their children and sleep beside their cots. Cicely had always encouraged this practice, believing that it was the best way to treat a child. If the mother was dead or sick, the family nearly always provided an aunt or someone else who would come in with the child. If treatment was going to take a long time, as it often did, the mother sometimes got bored and wanted to go home. She would generally come and tell Cicely that her own mother was sick or she must go home and plant her cultivation. Cicely always replied, "All right, you have paid five shillings for treatment in the hospital, but that only applies if you wait until the hospital treatment is finished. If you go out now I am afraid it will cost you five pounds." But no matter how long the child had to stay in hospital the charge was never increased as long as the mother did what she was asked to do, which was to stay in hospital with the child until the child was well. Sometimes the mother would go home if she knew the child was happy and doing well, but she would come back later and take the child home again; and she nearly always left an older sister of the child or another close relative.

To make life more comfortable for the mothers, Cicely persuaded the Government to build what was generally known as a "cowshed", a room where the mothers could keep their own things and wash, cook and relax. Here they could see their relatives and gossip. Cicely realised that they also passed on a good deal of health education to each other.

She began to make nightly visits to the mothers, and make friends with them in the hope that they would gradually feel able to talk to her about unmentionable things.

As she came to know them better she realised that some mothers very much wanted to talk to her. They would begin to do this when there were few people about. Perhaps they would call her into a corner to ask whether she had noticed such and such and what did she really think. Gradually she gained their confidence, and was able to explain that this was a sickness that she didn't understand and that they might help her to find out all about it and save some of the other children.

After many conversations that carefully skirted the real

points at issue and an infinite variety of unvoiced communications, she realised that the mothers had no real objection to post-mortems. It wasn't against their religion, which seemed to demand only that the body should be buried in its home compound on the day the child died. But why, then, did the mothers hurry away from the hospital with the dying children strapped to their backs?

She learnt the answer late one night, talking to a friendly mammy, tiny, bright and shrivelled, whose fourth child was dying from the mystery disease.

"Why do they do it?" asked Cicely quietly. "Why do they run away with their dying babies?"

"The answer is simple." The woman stared wistfully towards the wards. Cicely waited in silence until she spoke again.

"On the bus you must pay much money for a corpse. We take them home before they die because the fare is less."

"Is that all?" cried Cicely, astonished, and unable to contain her excitement.

"That is all. It costs much money."

"Good God, it's so simple. Why didn't I think of it before?"

She began to say to mothers, "Leave the child in peace until it is dead. Let it die in comfort if it's going to die. And if you will allow me to make an examination I will pay the bus fare." And she would add, "I guarantee to give you the death certificate and let you get away as quickly as possible. I won't keep you waiting if you want to go home and bury the child on the same day."

She realised that, approached in the right way, nearly every mother would give permission for a post-mortem examination.

Armed with what she had discovered she returned to O'Hara May, trying not to appear too triumphant.

"O.K." he said. "Go ahead and do your bloody P.M.'s. But as a matter of interest, are you proposing to cut up corpses in the bathroom?"

"I'm glad you've mentioned the bathroom." She was cool now that her object was achieved. "Do you realise, Dr O'Hara

May, that the bathroom is the only place in the hospital where we can put a dead body? It's most unhealthy."

He laughed. "Cicely, I'm devoted to you, but I never knew anyone so quick to exploit a situation. I promise that I will look into the question of a mortuary. Perhaps in ten years' time they'll build you one!"

"I'm going to beat this disease before then," said Cicely with determination.

"Don't think that a few autopsy reports are going to give you the answer."

"I don't. But like Father Brown, I believe that you can't find a solution until you find the problem. The only way to do that is to get the pathology straight."

She was now free to do post-mortems, but organising them was even more difficult than she had anticipated. If they were going to be done at all, it must be quickly. By custom and religion the body had to be buried in its own home compound before sunset. She knew that the goodwill of the mothers depended on her respecting this. Another reason for performing the examination immediately after death was the speed with which a dead body decomposes in African heat.

But Dr O'Hara May's joke about the bathroom was not irrelevant. The bodies had to be put there because there was nowhere else. But it was inconceivable that messy operations could be done there.

If she was going to discover anything of value the examinations would have to be done in a properly equipped post-mortem room, preferably near a laboratory with facilities for staining slides, looking down microscopes and doing chemical investigations.

Another difficulty was to find children who were suffering from this disease alone, for it was rare to find a seriously sick child who did not also have yaws and scabies and malaria and worms, and perhaps bronchitis or pneumonia as well. These other diseases complicated her observations. But she had kept careful notes for many months, and she now made up her mind that whenever she came across a case that seemed wholly or chiefly due to this mysterious disease she would, no matter what the cost or the inconvenience, immediately take the body personally to the hospital at Korle Bu two miles away and do a full post-mortem examination. She knew that this was the only practical way to solve the problem.

She carried out this resolution despite considerable inconvenience. Sometimes in the middle of a busy out-patients clinic, with a hundred or more patients waiting to be seen, a child would die. She would put the corpse into the back of her car and drive to Korle Bu. There she did the post-mortem and the necessary tests, arranged the body carefully afterwards, drove back and gave the parents the death certificate and also, from her own salary, the fare to go home with the corpse on the bus. It was time-consuming and emotionally exhausting and distressing, but she persisted with a doggedness that sprang from her profound belief in the value of what she was doing.

"And what have you found?" asked O'Hara May one day.

"It's a strange disease," Cicely said. "But there's one constant pathological finding. In every post-mortem I've done I've found a fatty liver."

"Is that all?"

"Yes. I know it doesn't sound much, but I think it's important. It suggests to me that they *are* all cases of the same disease, but not an infection. My hunch is that it's due to faulty diet."

"Perhaps it's some form of pellagra?"

"No," she said, emphatically. "That's different."

"Do you think that other people will dismiss it as pellagra?"

"They may well," she said, and added with feeling, "especially if they don't know what they are talking about. I'm sure that our whole concept of food and disease is wrong. Because vitamins were discovered a few years ago we've all gone vitamin mad and can only think of nutritional disease in terms of them."

"What do you propose to do?"

"I've learnt so much from talking to Africans that I think I'll carry on with the same method."

His answer betrayed his doubt. "If you believe that talking to

African women will lead to important scientific discovery, good luck to you. I'm sure those learned professors in Cambridge will be agog for news."

Cicely laughed. "You bet they will. I shouldn't think they've even heard of the Gold Coast, let alone its diseases. And they don't care either."

"You're right," he said sadly. "I'm afraid that whatever momentous discovery you make, no one at home will sit up and say, 'Ha, news from the Gold Coast'."

"What exactly do you give the child to eat?" Cicely had learnt to ask the question in Ga and Twi and several other African languages, and she was becoming more skilled at understanding what the mothers said although they were often rambling and indirect. She felt sure that here was the answer. There was something wrong with the feeding of these children, and this caused, or at least contributed to, this disease.

Ghanaian customs in feeding young children were poor by European standards. When the baby needed more than the mother's breast it was usual to give some form of maize. Many children seemed to be reasonably healthy on this diet, but many were not. Cicely began to make an intensive study of the lives and eating habits of the sick children compared with the healthy ones.

She believed implicitly that the best way to treat disease is to prevent it, and the best way to prevent it is to care for every family and not just for the sick ones. She knew that much serious disease could be avoided in this way. There were few general practitioners in Ghana at that time. Children were rarely taken to hospital, and the high mortality rate among the babies and children was accepted as part of normal life. Yet she knew that many African women were anxious to bring their children for treatment.

She was determined to care for the healthy children as well as those who were ill. But one of the problems was the queuing. When a woman brings a healthy child and finds fifty people with sick babies waiting, she doesn't see the point of joining the queue just for supervision. Cicely decided that the best way to encourage mothers to bring their healthy babies would be to organise a large number of "well baby clinics" in different parts of the town, run by nurses from the hospital and by health visitors. Within a year she had organised fifteen of these centres in Accra. She also studied the best time of day to hold the clinics to make it easy for the mothers, and chose 7 to 9 in the mornings or 5 to 7 in the evenings, when the fathers were at home. She didn't bother much about the building. She would find someone to lend a room, perhaps a garage, an empty shop or the verandah of a school. At first the nurses would visit in the area. They saw the children who had been in hospital and needed supervision after returning home. They also visited newborn babies. They would advise the families and talk to them in the home about follow-up treatment. If they found a child who was seriously sick they had to write on the card and tell the mother to bring it to see Cicely next morning at the hospital. They treated minor illnesses themselves, and persuaded as many mothers as possible to bring their children to the healthy babies' centre. Every nurse in the hospital was attached to a centre and went out carrying scales and a small box of simple drugs including quinine, cough mixture and ointment for scabies. They did not charge for treatment, but they were not allowed to give the patients medicine to take home. If this was needed the patient had to visit Cicely at the hospital.

One of the first visible results of this new way of organising the medical services struck Cicely as rather funny. In one year the attendances at the out-patients department of the Marie Louise Hospital fell from 30,000 to 26,000. Immediately she received a letter from the authorities wanting to know why. It was signed by a high official of the Medical Services. Cicely wrote pointing out that they already had 15,000 attendances at the "well baby clinics" in the first year, and that these had included many children suffering from minor diseases who would otherwise have attended the out-patients department. It amused her to think that Headquarters felt that this needed investigation.

At first she regarded the matter lightheartedly. But the medical official thought otherwise. He was renowned for his self-esteem and his love of order in the English fashion, and he was not satisfied with the state of affairs at the Princess Marie Louise Hospital. He sent for Cicely.

She found him sitting in a big leather chair, and thought he looked like an angry pigeon. But for the first time she realised that it might be serious, especially as Dr O'Hara May was away.

"I have sent for you, Dr Williams," he said, as though addressing a meeting, "because I am not satisfied with the report from the Princess Marie Louise Hospital. I am also not satisfied with your reply to my letter."

"I'm sorry. I thought I had made it clear."

"Very clear," he said, sarcastically. "Very clear that you are not doing what you are supposed to do."

"What do you mean?" Cicely smiled deliberately to keep her temper.

"You are supposed to be preventing disease in this town. You are supposed to be conducting Infant Welfare Centres on the same lines as in England. That means seeing well infants in the Welfare Clinic and sick ones at the hospital."

"No." She felt the blood of rage rush up her neck and added "sir," in an attempt to control herself. "It isn't like that. It can't be on the same lines as in England. Infant welfare clinics were introduced there to fill the gaps between general practitioner and hospital. Out here there are practically no general practitioners, and most Africans wouldn't think of taking their children to hospital. Most of the children we see here are sick by European standards. You can't separate the sheep from the goats."

The medical official looked at his fingernails and then over his spectacles.

"If the children are sick they should be referred to the hospital in the customary way." He turned away as though that was all he had to say.

"That would be impossible," cried Cicely. "First of all

the mothers won't bring them unless we make it easy for them. Most of them don't regard their children as sick because all the children they know are just as bad. What's more, if all the sick ones did come to the hospital we couldn't cope with them. We shouldn't have anything like enough staff."

"Nevertheless," he said stiffly, "I deplore the fall in attendances." There was a typewritten sheet of figures in front of him and he was twirling a bunch of keys. "It looks bad," he muttered, "very bad."

"In Whitehall?" asked Cicely, pertly. She was angry now and past caring. He looked up sharply.

"Yes, in Whitehall, if you put it that way. I should like to remind you, Dr Williams, that it is Whitehall to whom you are answerable. In my view you are deliberately disobeying your orders, which are to organise the medical services so that the Africans may benefit from the English system of child care."

"English system fiddlesticks." Cicely snapped her fingers in temper. "First of all it's totally unsuitable for Africa, and secondly, in my opinion, it's unsuitable in England too. The separation of preventive and curative aspects of child health work in England was due to an historical accident, and it was a most unfortunate mistake. We're saddled with it now at home with all its disastrous consequences. But for God's sake let's not inflict it on the Africans."

She stalked out of the office and out of the building recognising the satisfaction of having let off steam over something she felt strongly about. But she soon regretted the lapse, and later she paid for it heavily.

She continued to search for the origins of the mysterious disease. She noticed that there was often something wrong in the child's background which might seem bizarre to a European.

"Are you the mother of this baby?"

"No, I am his grandmother. His mother is dead."

"How is the baby fed?"

"With breast milk."

"Who feeds the baby?"

"I do."

"But you are his grandmother. Have you milk?"

"Yes, a little. Not as much as his mother would have. I do my best. His mother is dead."

"How old is your own youngest child?"

"I do not know her age. She was the mother of this baby. It was her first. But I still have milk."

This child was very sick indeed, and would soon be dead. Cicely took him into hospital and fed him on varied food containing much meat and fish. To her surprise he improved rapidly and recovered. So did others like him. But some died, and she came to the conclusion that by the time they were admitted to hospital the disease was too often irreversible.

But other children died too, even some whom she had seen in out-patients before they were sick enough to be admitted to hospital. She took trouble to explain to the mothers the principles of good diet, and sent nurses to the patients' houses to make sure that the food was available. Yet still some of the children died. In the case of one of them Cicely had proof that the mother had ignored her instructions. But with the others it was impossible to tell.

"I'm confused and worried," she said to O'Hara May when he returned from leave. "I feel I'm on the brink of finding the answer, yet I'm not sure what to do next."

"Never mind. I want you to write a description of the disease and I'll include it in my annual report, and perhaps other people who have seen the disease will be able to give us some more information about it."

Cicely wrote an article called *A Nutrition Disease of Childhood* describing everything that she had observed. It was published in the Gold Coast Medical Report of 1932–33, but it produced no response.

On her next home leave she took with her the photographs and records that she had collected about the disease.

"Who on earth do you expect to read the report?" asked Dr Helen Mackay, her former chief at the Queen Elizabeth

Hospital in Hackney. "You should publish it where people will read it."

"I can't," said Cicely, helplessly. "I don't know anything about the disease."

"Rubbish," said Dr Mackay. "Publish."

A few days later Cicely took her article to the offices of the *Archives of Disease in Childhood*, the most important journal in Britain concerned with diseases of children. The editor leant back in his chair, flipped the pages of the typescript and said, "I can't publish this. No one's interested in the Gold Coast."

Under Dr Mackay's influence the editor changed his mind, and the article was published under the title *A Nutrition Disease of Children associated with a Maize Diet*. It produced only letters from a doctor in Nyasaland saying that she was obviously describing cases of pellagra which she had failed to diagnose. She was certain that he was wrong, and there the matter rested. Back in Accra she wrote to Dr Mackay, "I must get proof that it really is a disease in its own right and that it is not cured by vitamins. Perhaps one day people will realise that it is not pellagra."

As she gained experience of the disease she began to recognise its earliest stages. Mothers brought babies who had just a slight swelling of their feet, and she realised that this was one of the first signs of the disease. The swelling probably developed because the legs hung down immobile as the child was carried on its mother's back. She told these mothers to come back in a week and gave them advice as to what the child should eat. She told them not to give the *akassa* by itself but to beat in an egg, use groundnut soup and try to buy some tinned milk. She also told them to use fish. She guessed that the condition was probably largely due to low protein diet. This turned out to be an inspired guess.

Some of the children recovered but others deteriorated. Cicely was not making much progress in her discussions with the Africans, neither mothers nor nurses. She had no means of measuring the children's food or of telling how much or how little her advice was responsible for the cases which recovered.

One day she became upset. During a single morning clinic at the Marie Louise Hospital she had to admit three children with the disease. Two of them were obviously dying, and one of these Cicely had already saved from death only two months before.

When she became distressed she tended to lose her temper. She turned in fury on her nurses and burst out, "Why do you let your children get into this state? This is your disease. It isn't my disease. Do you really not know what it is?"

One of the nurses was called Christine Bryant. Cicely's outburst seemed to penetrate her usual imperturbability. She looked Cicely straight in the face and said, "Yes, doctor, we know what the sickness is. It is *kwashiorkor*."

"What does *kwashiorkor* mean?"

"It means the sickness that the older child gets when the next baby is born."

"My God," said Cicely, half to herself. "I believe that's the explanation."

"Please, doctor?" said the nurse anxiously.

"I was thinking of the psalm," said Cicely. "'*I will refrain my soul and keep it low like a child that is weaned from his mother. Yea my soul is even as a weaned child*'."

Excitedly she talked to O'Hara May. "I am convinced that the weanling children in this country are not getting enough protein to eat. Everything I've seen fits the picture. Whether or not they recover depends partly on how far the disease has progressed and partly on how far the mother is prepared to alter the child's diet. She is less likely to do this if she is occupied with a new baby, and that's why it's called *kwashiorkor*, the weanling disease."

Soon after this she received a letter from the editor of *The Lancet* asking her to write an article about the disease. After it was published she was again reprimanded for failing to diagnose pellagra, and again she knew that the accusation was wrong but had no concrete means of refuting it. But a few years later she went, at her own expense, to New Orleans, because there had been many cases of pellagra in that town which had been studied by Dr Joseph Goldberger at the Charity Hospital.

There she was able to study the disease and to show conclusively that it was not the same as *kwashiorkor*. Later, when suitable chemical tests became widely available, it was also shown that, as she had predicted, cases of *kwashiorkor* were deficient in blood protein.

But Cicely herself could not take part in these discoveries which showed how millions of children's lives could be saved. For by that time she was far from Africa. Events had overwhelmed her, and she was experiencing malnutrition at first hand at the limits of human endurance.

Cicely had realised early that advances in medicine are only sometimes due to discoveries, and that improved methods of treatment may be merely a question of common sense. Sometimes it was so absurdly simple that she felt ashamed of not achieving more. On one of her first excursions with a nurse to visit in the homes she found a buxom young mother with her first baby about a week old and starving. The mother had engorged breasts, but her nipples were not sufficiently developed for the baby to get the milk. Clearly it would die unless something was done. There was no spoon in the house, but she managed to buy one from a local shop. She showed the mother how to express the milk into the spoon and feed the baby with it. "It was the simplest thing," she wrote to her own mother in Jamaica, "but without our explanation and demonstration that baby would certainly have died of starvation. This kind of thing often happens. Sometimes such things are so simple that it makes me want to cry."

But sometimes enthusiasm overcame common sense, particularly concerning personal safety. For instance, in those days, before penicillin or prontosil, it was dangerous to do post-mortems with even the smallest unprotected cut on one's hand. One of the worst germs that could be picked up in this way was the haemolytic streptococcus, which was rampant, virulent and often fatal. One day a child came into hospital and died almost immediately. Cicely did a post-mortem, found nothing specific, but sent some blood for culture. Next day she was sick herself from a small scratch on a finger. The swelling reached as far as her left ear and she had much pain. She was taken to hospital delirious with fever. Two days later she received the laboratory report on the blood specimen from the child. It had died with infection from the dreaded haemolytic streptococcus.

She now knew that she was in grave personal danger, but she still felt unable to make a fuss or to betray her anxiety.

"I may have picked up something from a post-mortem," she said diffidently to the doctor.

"Nonsense, my dear girl. If that were so you'd be in the mortuary by now."

She suppressed her thoughts and fear and concentrated on survival. The infection subsided. When the swelling was confined to the left arm she insisted on going back to work. But when it began to fluctuate she became nervous again and returned to the hospital. The doctor aspirated some pus and sent it for culture. Two days later he telephoned her.

"Do you know what they found in that pus? A haemolytic streptococcus! You must come back to hospital instantly and have it cleaned out."

"I've had it for three weeks," said Cicely belligerently. "I'm busy. There are a hundred patients waiting to see me."

There was an explosive noise on the line.

"Now. At once. I'm scrubbed up and waiting for you."

Twenty-five minutes later she was on the operating table. She was seriously ill after the operation, but the "clean out" probably saved her life. Since treatment for this illness was rarely successful there was a good deal of anxiety about her.

While she was recovering her old friend John Ferrers, the administrative officer, came to see her. He found her sitting up in bed writing a paper on *kwashiorkor.*

"Only when I'm ill do I have time to be creative."

"I heard you were at death's door."

"I always enjoy going sick. It's marvellous. Between you and me, John, if I had the courage I would malinger as much as possible."

Gradually her health returned. Back in her own bungalow

she strengthened her muscles by digging in her garden. All day mammies walked along the Dodoma road beside the garden. When they saw her digging they would call out in cheerful voices, "Ayko, awura" ("Well done"). Cicely was pleased that she could now give the correct reply, for it takes years for a European to learn a tone language. She had now been in Africa for more than four years, and felt very much part of it.

She returned to work before she was fit, and was immediately precipitated into an unpleasant experience.

"Where is Jacques?" she asked, as she entered one of the wards. Jacques was a small boy, the son of a French father and an African mother. He was a particular favourite of Cicely's, partly because of his engaging manner and partly because he had been in hospital for so long that he seemed to be part of it. He had tuberculous peritonitis, a non-infectious form of tuberculosis. She felt sure that she would be able to cure him in the end, even if he had to stay in hospital for several years. She knew that if he went home he would not receive the care that was necessary.

The ward sister drew her attention to another patient, a lively little girl who was jumping about at the bottom of the next cot.

"Where's Jacques?" Cicely repeated, suddenly afraid that while she was away Jacques had gone downhill and died. She knew that the standard of care that the patients received deteriorated when she did not supervise the details.

"He was discharged, Doctor."

"Discharged?" She found this difficult to believe. The medical officer who had looked after the Children's Hospital while she was ill had visited her in hospital, and she had specifically explained to him about Jacques and how it was most important that the child should remain in hospital. "Did his mother take him away?"

"No, Doctor. The fat doctor from Health Department came. He say no infectious cases allowed."

"But Jacques isn't infectious."

"He say patients with tuberculosis not allowed in hospital."

"But there's nowhere else for them to go." Cicely was angry. She realised that the "fat doctor" was her old enemy of the medical administration. He was now in charge again because O'Hara May had been recalled to England. This was Cicely's punishment for being rude about the organisation of child care.

"It's monstrous. I'm in charge here. Even if I'm ill he can't come and discharge my patients."

"That's what he did, Doctor."

"I have the address of the child. I shall go and fetch him back myself. He'll die if he's left outside."

In her office was a pile of mail, including a letter from the official himself instructing her not to admit any more children with tuberculosis to the ward.

She knew in her heart that he was acting within his rights, and this made the injustice even harder to bear. In her first free moment she visited the child's home. Jacques was markedly worse. His belly was swollen with fluid. He half recognised her through staring, sunken eyes. She tried to persuade his mother to bring him back to hospital. She resented deeply what had happened and was willing, even anxious, to disobey her orders.

But the mother wished to keep the child at home. She said that he was going to die anyway, and Cicely could not but agree with her.

Then started a long and distressing correspondence with the official concerned. He refused to give way, and repeated his instructions that she was not to admit cases of tuberculosis. She ignored these instructions and deliberately admitted more cases of T.B. She received another letter saying that the instructions must be loyally observed. Her reply was that her first loyalty was to her patients.

Tired, sick and discouraged, she determined to make every effort to be transferred to another position in the Colonial Service.

She had now been in the colony for five years, and Government regulations stated that at the end of this time one was entitled to extra leave for study. She applied for this but was refused. Because of her recent experiences, she insisted that aspersions had been cast on her knowledge of tuberculosis, and she asked to be allowed to go to England to study the subject. Finally she received a two months' extension of leave, and decided to spend it in preparing for the Membership Examination of the Royal College of Physicians. The failure rate was high, but if she could pass she would be in a strong position for a specialist appointment.

She did a short preparatory course at the Charing Cross Hospital, but never took the examination. Two days beforehand, she received a welcome letter informing her that she was to be given the membership because of the work she had already published. This was a great honour.

Although she now had her membership she was not surprised, when she returned to the Gold Coast, to find that she had been rusticated from Accra and posted to Kumasi. This meant that she would not be promoted to a specialist job or to a permanent posting in Accra. It also meant an end to her hopes of building up a children's unit in the Princess Marie Louise Hospital.

In spite of her disappointment she wrote cheerfully to her mother, "The work in Ashanti will have many compensations. For one thing there is a maternity ward as well as a children's ward in the Kumasi clinic. There is also an enormous out-patients department and about twelve well-established 'weighing centres' in different parts of the town. I shall have the opportunity to do something that I've wanted to do for a long time, which is to make a proper study of the pattern of child health and disease in the Gold Coast. This is very much needed. I shall certainly see an enormous amount of clinical material, and I shall be able to compare conditions in Ashanti with those in Accra."

CHAPTER IV

THE MORE CICELY thought about it, the more pleased she was with her appointment in Kumasi. It did not lessen the pain and disappointment of the whole miserable affair, but it was some compensation. She had lost a chance to build up the children's unit in Accra, but she now had the opportunity to do something else that might, in the end, be even more valuable.

Ever since she had first arrived in Koforidua five years before she had realised that there was a big need for a survey of sickness and health among children in the Gold Coast. The lack of the knowledge that such a survey could provide impaired the value of children's medical and child care services. For years now she had been collecting material and keeping careful notes. She was always hoping to complete the study and write it up, first of all in the form of a doctorate thesis for the University of Oxford, and then possibly as a book which would become a standard work. This would be an immensely satisfying achievement and might turn her disgrace in Accra into a blessing.

With her experience and her knowledge of Twi she was now in a strong position to study diseases as they existed, and the social, economic and nutritional background which produced them.

She was particularly interested in studying the attitudes of parents towards children, for she believed that this was the background to the pattern of health and disease. Increasingly she was impressed with the quality of family life in Ghana. Ghanaian mothers were exceptionally devoted to their children. But since only about half of all the children born alive survived to maturity, it was taken for granted that a number of them would die. Death and disease were attributed to the evil eye or to the influence of witches or to bad luck which followed you because you walked on the wrong side of the road or outraged some particular tradition. But Cicely found that once she had their confidence many of the mothers carried out her instructions diligently. They began to understand that she was trying to help their children, and they saw that her methods were good. Many of the women were remarkably quick in the way they accepted, absorbed and followed her teaching. She could feel them learning that a tummy upset was due to dietetic indiscretion rather than to malevolent glances of the evil eye; that some features in a child's growth and development could not be prevented or cured by medication; and that there was much that was within their own control. Cicely felt that she was making progress.

She came across a curious form of child care among the so-called "fetish" children. If several children had died in a family, which was not unusual, the next child was sometimes dedicated to a "fetish", which was a local cult, usually under some form of village deity. Such a child was brought up to look unkempt and neglected. Its hair was not combed and it was dressed in rags. These children were often wild and badly behaved, and were given disparaging names such as "We laugh at death", "It doesn't matter" or "Nobody wants her". If the child did survive ransom was paid to the "fetish", or, if it was a girl, she had to be bought back from the "fetish" before she could be given in marriage or the father accept a bride price. Cicely watched the growth of many of these "fetish" children. Many of them did survive, and a great transformation took place when their hair was cut and they assumed the ordinary conventions of the local adolescents.

One day a woman came with a baby of two or three days old and already starving. The woman said that she had no milk. This was unusual, because African women lactate magnificently. Cicely had never before seen a mother in Ghana who lacked milk for her baby. She examined the woman's breasts, and found that what she said was true. Cicely arranged for her to come into hospital to learn how to use tinned milk. There was no question of fresh milk, for there were no cows and goats were never milked. She discovered how much the woman could afford to pay, and tried to organise the baby's diet accordingly. She had already discovered that there were no relatives prepared to wet-nurse the baby. As soon as the artificial feeds were started the baby began to do well. One night Cicely was doing the night round in the ward and discovered that the woman was awake and obviously waiting to see her. She said that she wanted to talk to her very particularly and that it was important. Cicely took her downstairs to her consulting room and the woman told her that this was very, very private indeed but she wanted her to know that the baby was not hers and that the real mother was dead.

"But why didn't you tell me this when you first came to see me?"

"If I had told you that it was not my baby you would have said, 'Take the baby home, you know it can't live'."

There was, Cicely found, a strong belief among the people that if the mother died her soul would come and call to the baby, who was bound to die too. So a motherless baby was given up as hopeless, and few even tried to help it to survive.

"You are wrong," said Cicely, half to herself, then added, "You were right to bring the baby to see me. Motherless babies do not die because the souls of their dead mothers call them. They die because they are not fed properly. This baby will live because I have taught you how to raise it."

"Legends such as these can change in a few years, especially if you demonstrate visibly that they are wrong." This was Cicely's intense belief, and the foundation of much of her work in Africa. When she returned to Kumasi in 1956, she found that there was now a whole ward full of motherless babies. Over a large part of the country, if a mother died the baby was brought at once to the Kumasi Hospital and left there for up to two years, properly fed, and then returned to its relatives. Everyone could now see that even an orphan child could survive, and the idea was now widely accepted. There was no more talk of the souls of dead mothers calling the babies.

Sometimes the solution was wet-nursing, but this involved the question of the ownership of a child, which was complicated. If a woman had given her breast to a child she had some claim on that child afterwards. If it was a girl she would have some claim to the bride price. In most cases Cicely found that people would not allow babies to be breast fed except by close relatives such as the sister of the mother, and if the mother had no sister with milk at the moment then it would probably be difficult to find anyone.

But she was continually impressed by the African women's powers of lactation. She found that it was not unusual for a grandmother to feed a child because its mother was dead. She saw a woman who had not had a baby for nineteen years breast feed her granddaughter because the mother had died, and she breast fed that child up to the age when it got *kwashiorkor*. She found many cases where the grandmother acted as a dummy, and often she had a little milk in her breasts and would contribute something towards the nutrition of the child. The women often lived in compounds together, and the child would run to any of the women in the family if he was distressed or upset.

At that time, when a woman was far on in pregnancy, she usually went to her mother's compound and was delivered there. Afterwards she prepared food for her husband, but did not live with him until the baby was at least a year old. Meanwhile the baby might be handed round and nursed by the grandmother or anyone else who had milk. If then settled down and was fed principally by the mother, but in moments of stress or if the mother was away it might be comforted or put to the breast by the grandmother or other close relatives.

Cicely already knew how greatly fertility was admired in Ghana. If she asked a mother how many children she had, she would include all the abortions and miscarriages. The antenatal clinics were just as popular as the ones Cicely had run on the coast. The women were so pleased to be pregnant that they would have come twice a week for the whole nine months if Cicely had permitted it. Enthusiasm for maternity, in fact, was so great that during the antenatal clinic there were usually several elderly optimists who would turn up and say, "I have been pregnant for six years. Please give me something to make my belly swell." The menopause was often a personal tragedy, because once they had passed the age of childbearing they were sometimes demoted from the wife class into the dowager class.

Among these women there were a few cases of pseudocyesis or hysterical false pregnancy. One woman was so convinced that she was pregnant that she had the profile of an advanced case of twins. Cicely had to take her into hospital and have many talks with her before she could persuade her that there was no baby there. Her waist measurement was enormous. She must have been maintaining a tremendous diaphragmatic pressure to achieve the figure that was suitable to her conviction that she was pregnant. Her exertions were affecting her heart, which was beating rapidly, but returned to normal when she overcame the delusion of pregnancy.

The Ghanaians were devoted parents. In seven years Cicely saw only two abandoned children. But there was a tendency to look after the youngest child at the expense of the older ones. She felt that it was generally accepted that toddlers were miserable, potbellied and spindle-legged, as though this was a stage through which children must pass, with many dying on the way. She felt sure that this legend could also be defeated by visible demonstration of its falsity.

During all her years in Africa she scarcely ever saw older children teasing younger ones. Little girls, and sometimes boys too, were often left in charge of smaller brothers and sisters, and Cicely was impressed by their consistently responsible attitude. She believed that this was one of the reasons why the girls made excellent nurses. They easily learnt to look after sick children, and also how to teach the mothers in the wards and in the outpatients; how to explain things to the mothers and make them feel at home in hospital; and how to adjudicate when the mothers quarrelled. Cicely found them inspiring to work with, not only because they were devoted to the work but because they were always urging her to do more.

Like Accra, Kumasi had a sort of family hospital. Children were admitted with their mothers or with other close relatives, and there was a "cowshed" where these relatives could keep their belongings and wash and gather and gossip. Cicely had good opportunities to talk to the mother and children, and she came to know them well. One day a new Sister came from England to take charge of a ward. She was impatient during Cicely's ward rounds because she took so long to finish and spent so much time talking to the mothers and the children. One child had been admitted alone because his mother was dead and there was no one to come in with him. He was about three years old, and needed treatment for worms. He was not crying, but he looked grim and unresponsive and was obviously horrified at being left there with strangers. Cicely sat down on the floor and explained to him that the following day he would have some medicine but until he had had it he could only have soup and milk, although the other children would be having rice and fish and bananas. Afterwards he would have nice fufu to eat and other food that he liked. The child sat with a scowl on his face. Sister stood tapping her scissors impatiently. When Cicely had finished she went back to her office, and not long afterwards Sister came and said, "I'll never be impatient with you again." There was a table in the children's ward with little chairs for the "up" patients. Sister had forgotten about the child's fluid diet, and had handed rice and fufu to the child. He had risen to his feet, pushed away the chair and walked out on to the verandah, and held on to the bars shaking his head from side to side.

"I find African children incredibly sensible and trustworthy," said Cicely. "I think it must be because they're with grownups so much and the grownups never talk down to them. They seem to be people in their own right from the start."

"There is a child outside on the verandah," said the Sister. "She looks about fourteen and she has been here ever since I came, which is nearly a fortnight. I don't know what to do about her. She sweeps the verandah and does any little job she can find. She arrives at dawn and hangs around all day, often until far in the night. Her one idea seems to be to help me and the patients. If she can't find anything to do she sits quietly in the corner just waiting for someone to take notice of her. I don't think she would go away, even if I had the heart to try to get rid of her."

Cicely went out on to the verandah and recognised the girl at once. She had come to the hospital a few weeks before because she was keen to train as a nurse. But there was no room for her. There were already more applicants than vacancies. Girls who had been through the training were much sought after as brides, and because of this high regard many were anxious to come and train at the maternal and child health centre. This girl's school qualifications were poor.

Cicely looked at her quizzically. The girl wriggled and reminded Cicely of a dog asking to be taken for a walk. But there was intelligence and steadiness in her eyes.

"All right, you win," she said. "We'll train you as a nurse."

The girl smiled, and it seemed to Cicely that after this the smile never left her face. For the rest of Cicely's time in Kumasi she felt that she was always followed by the young nurse's smile. Despite lack of schooling she made an excellent nurse, and Cicely never regretted her sudden decision.

During one night round she found the ward overcrowded, and could scarcely pick her way between the mothers on the floor and the children in the cots and beds. This was disturbing, because next day there would be urgent cases to admit. She started to discuss with the night nurse which patients it might be possible to discharge next day.

"Who is in that cot?"

"The baby we admitted today, Doctor."

"Who is that on the floor?"

"That is the mother of the baby."

"And who is that beside the mother?"

"That is the mother of the mother, Doctor, and she has also come in."

"This really is a bit much," said Cicely crossly. She went across the room, woke the grandmother and said sarcastically, "Why didn't you bring your mother into hospital with you as well?"

"Oh," said the woman, rubbing her eyes, "she's at home with a new baby."

Afterwards it occurred to Cicely that this was probably true. The mother was about fourteen and the grandmother was under thirty, which probably made the great-grandmother about forty-two.

Every sixth Sunday in Kumasi a day was celebrated which was called *Kwesi adei*. The local chiefs came to town with their followers and drummers and paid homage to the Kumasihene, the king of Kumasi. Cicely loved pomp and pageantry, and found these occasions enthralling because the procession went right through the town and some of the chiefs were carried in litters covered in lion or leopard skins. The chiefs were dressed in multi-coloured robes, often of woven Kinti cloths. Many of them wore gold headdresses, and sometimes black velvet bands round their heads with big bosses of gold. Each had an enormous umbrella of state, often of gorgeous silk or brocade, which was carried by a man who twirled or tossed it as he walked along. The women dressed in their most decorative clothes, scraped their hair back and usually plastered it with motor grease over a coconut shell, making a high sort of pompadour style, set with large gold ornaments. Each chief was accompanied by his official stool, which was the sign of authority. Some chiefs had many followers, gorgeously dressed. Long hollow tree trunks were carried on the heads of two men walking in line, and the drummer walked behind them, drumming on the end of the drum. They marched to the palace and there were songs and dances and feasting.

If an important person died there was a big funeral. In the old days it had been a yam festival, which was rather like Harvest Festival. In Ga it was called the *homowa*, which means "we laugh at hunger". But the yam festival was accompanied by human sacrifice, and this was eventually stopped. Even so, there were moments of uneasiness. In her last year in Kumasi there was a celebration when the yam festival was again permitted. Cicely felt certain that human sacrifices were taking place. Her patients dropped from about 200 a day down to twenty, and many people were afraid to go out. One evening, at the height of the celebration, in order to drive from her bungalow to the hospital she had to pass the mausoleum of the Kings of Ashanti. It was her usual time between 10 and 11 o'clock in the evening. As she passed she saw three lorries parked outside the mausoleum. She drove past them, and one of the lorries followed her and waited outside the hospital while she was inside. She came home by a different route so as not to pass the mausoleum again. She felt that someone was watching her all the time to make quite certain that she was out of the way. Later her nurses and other people whispered to her the reason—fear of human sacrifice.

Christianity as well as paganism was strong in West Africa, for missionaries were everywhere. Thousands of people went to church on Sunday and observed non-Christian ceremonies on other occasions. At moments of stress they would do everything they could to ensure better fate or better luck. All the Christian denominations insisted on monogamy, which was not easy in West Africa, and was often used for private marital purposes. If a man was tired of his wives he would sometimes join a religious sect or a Christian community, just to get rid of them. If he acquired more wives later, he would again change his denomination and do the same again. Cicely thought that the Salvation Army was particularly sensible in dealing with this. They said that if a man had wives and wished to join the Salvation Army, he could do so but must continue to take good care of all his wives and he must not acquire more because, although monogamy was the ideal, joining a Christian body did not mean that he could neglect existing responsibilities.

She became increasingly concerned about the "fetishes". Many people on the Coast and in Ashanti belonged to them, and, whether Christians or not, were profoundly influenced by them. This involved ideas about spirits or supreme power that often conflicted with what Cicely was trying to do. She felt that the best way she could help her patients was to try to link what she was doing for them to a growing sense of personal responsibility. But the fetishes seemed to be a means by which people protected themselves from feelings of responsibility. To her the worst thing about the religious atmosphere of the country was its fatalism. People would be content to say that something had happened because of a witch, the evil eye or thunder, and this was an excuse not to do anything about it. Sometimes the fetishes were cruel, and they played a big part in the ideas of the people. "Even their Christianity is adapted to suit their fatalism," she wrote to her mother. "Only this morning I saw a child with a portrait of John Wesley hung round his neck as a charm against the evil eye. All the children come with charms. Often it is black powder in a small bottle tied round the neck. The most usual selection is a lion's claw, a lizard's jaw bone, the Sacred Heart, and a couple of saints for good measure."

"You can't do anything about the fatalism," she was told by Government officers with many more years of experience than she. "It's bred in them. If you want to achieve anything you have to do things to them. It's no good thinking they'll do things for themselves."

But she did not agree, and did not hesitate to speak her mind.

"I think that's wrong. I believe that this appalling fatalism, and also the power that the fetishes have over people, is due partly to ignorance and partly to lack of confidence. I am convinced that whenever one can show clearly that certain events are the result of certain forms of behaviour, then the fatalistic attitude diminishes. I believe that if we can teach the mothers to associate certain diseases with what they have done or not done, they will no longer be frightened of witchcraft or thunderbolts."

She set out to prove her point, slowly and arduously, and gradually the mothers came to realise that children could be protected more effectively from smallpox by vaccination than by wearing charms, and that if they fed their children in the way Cicely told them they did not develop the *kwashiorkor* disease.

The question of native medicine was always present. Some of the children would come in smeared from top to toe with noxious mixtures, and many parents would not bring a child to the "white man's hospital" until they were desperate and had tried every available form of native medicine.

"In the days before the missionaries," one of her African friends had told her during a long chat in Accra, "there were two separate professions in the African way of life. One was the priest of the local cult or fetish, and the other was the herbalist or doctor. But every now and then the herb doctor or 'witch' doctor had to perform a ceremony where, in accordance with the rules of his guild, he had to go round the house naming all the materials which he used for making up his drugs or ointments or enemas. When the missionaries came they thought that this was a bit of juju and they lumped the herbalist and the fetish priest together in one category. As a result, some of them got mixed up and started to practise the more obscure arts as well as their herbalism."

She saw some disastrous results of native medicine. A mother might give her child an enema containing something acutely irritating, or put some damaging drops into its eyes so that its sight was lost as a result of the treatment rather than the disease. Sometimes a case of obstructed labour was sent in with the perineum dangerously torn and pouring ghastly foul stuff that had been poked in. Cicely was also horrified by the fondness of the Africans for enemas. In some families each child had an enema every day, and as a result many children came in with prolapsed rectum and anal fissure, which had often been treated already with damaging concoctions.

Whenever a mother brought a child to see her Cicely always told her that while it was being treated by her it must not be given any other kind of medicine. But she gradually discovered that not all native medicine was harmful or even useless. Each form of treatment had to be considered on its own. Some of it was appalling, but some of it was better than anything that European medicine could provide. If she thought a patient suffered from some disease that the local witch doctors could treat better than she could, she would send the patients to the witch doctors. She would even pay the fee herself rather than let the child go without.

She gradually realised that the African witch doctors had some remarkable powers. She was amazed to discover that they had a successful treatment for tetanus, a disease for which European medicine could do nothing. There were many cases of tetanus in newborn babies because they were born in their homes, often under filthy conditions. The baby was usually delivered by its grandmother, who had no idea of asepsis, and infection entered through the umbilical cord, which had been cut with a dirty knife on the dirty floor. Sometimes Cicely had as many as five babies in the ward with tetanus, and they nearly always died.

One day a woman came from some distance with a baby about two weeks old, a severe case of tetanus. Cicely gave the best treatment then available. At the end of the week the baby's grandmother asked whether he was going to recover, and Cicely said frankly there was little hope.

"Would you mind if I took him to one of our own doctors?"

"Not at all. You have done everything I told you. You have done your best and I have tried my best. When the baby dies come back and I will give you the death certificate, because I know exactly what is wrong with it."

A few days later Cicely was in the ward with Amelia Kennedy, her senior African nurse.

"They haven't come back for the death certificate for that baby," she said.

"No, doctor. It is not yet dead."

Cicely was astonished. "But it was dying when it went out."

"No. The grandmother is a friend of mine and I saw the baby yesterday. He is getting better."

"Impossible!"

"But I've seen it."

"Where is the baby?"

"Being treated by one of our doctors called Ofole."

"I should like to meet him."

"I will take you this afternoon."

At the witch doctor's compound they were met by Ofole himself, a tall, middle-aged African, neat, bald and dignified, not at all the usual type of flashy witch doctor. Cicely explained why she had come and asked to see the child.

"Willingly." He led the way to the baby who was lying on a mattress in a corner, watched by his mother. Cicely drew back the covers and could scarcely believe what she saw.

At first she thought that it was a different child, but then she realised that there was no doubt because of a small birthmark on its leg. Yet the muscular spasm had gone and so had the arched back that, in Cicely's experience, always heralded death. The child lay quietly, curled normally. It opened its mouth, and its mother squeezed a few drops of milk into it.

"It is recovering," said Cicely. "Amazing!" Ofole smiled politely. She shook his hand enthusiastically. "This is tremendously important. In Europe we know nothing about it. Will you tell me what you have used to cure the baby?"

"Perhaps one day I will tell you."

She was longing to question him further but judged the moment inopportune, and concentrated on enthusiasm and polite formalities.

The following week she sent him another baby with advanced tetanus, and again he was successful. He was still polite, but he still refused to disclose his methods. After that she sent him all her cases of tetanus because she knew that this was the babies' only chance of survival. She discovered that he could also cure hopeless cases of meningitis which she knew would die if they stayed in the European hospital. These included proven cases of pneumococcal meningitis, a universally fatal disease. It seemed incredible. Cicely became more and more excited and anxious to discover the African's secrets.

She cultivated friendship with the witch doctor Ofole, and managed to scrape acquaintance with others. She discovered that in their treatment of tetanus they were using some substance that relaxed the spasm in the muscules without producing paralysis. This was the sort of drug that European doctors had been seeking for years without successs. She often went to the witch doctors' compound to see what they were using, and invited them to come to her own hospital. Ofole liked to come round her wards and she showed him her cases and told him exactly how she was treating them. Sometimes she tried making speeches to him.

"You can go to my country and you can learn everything that we know about medicine. It is part of our religion. We cannot hold back anything that is good for treating sick people."

Ofole gave his polite inscrutable smile. "Perhaps one day I will tell you."

And so it went on for three years.

One day she was working late in her office. It was dark in the corridor, and the only noise was the distant chatter of mothers in the "cowshed". Suddenly she jumped. The door swung open and framed the figure of Ofole. Behind him two small boys carried a sheet. Ofole bowed respectfully.

"I have come to show you my secrets." He sat down on the floor. The boys squatted beside him and he opened the sheet under the ceiling light. In it was a pile of different objects. Cicely could see roots and leaves and bark and dead cockroaches and bits of glass and dried lizards and many other things that she could not identify.

"Now I will tell you," he said, picking up a lizard's tail. Cicely seized the pen from her desk and a thick pad of paper and began to write down as much as possible of what he said. He took each of the contents of his sheet separately, talked about it and then handed it to Cicely. "And we take this and this and this and we pound them up and we put that on top of the head. And this and this and this we take and we use for an enema. And this and this we use for a drink. And this and this we use for a bath."

When the sheet was empty he folded it carefully, put it under his arm, stood up, bowed and departed back through the door, followed by the boys.

Cicely's hand still ached as she went back through her pages. She had been so busy writing that she had not really thought about what he actually said. But as she slowly deciphered the scribble an intense feeling of excitement rose in her. She realised that she now possessed knowledge that was new for Europeans, a type of knowledge with which Western medicine had as yet made no contact. Through the treatment of previously untreatable diseases it could lead to the saving of countless lives and the relief of untold suffering. Its further possibilities were limitless. Linked to European knowledge and traditions it could give rise to a whole new branch of medical thought. For Europeans, tetanus and pneumococcal meningitis were fatal and untreatable. Yet Ofole could cure them. She had seen him do it many times. Presumably she would now be able to do the same, and having learnt the method herself would be able to teach others.

She determined to learn the new method thoroughly, but she could not identify some of the things that Ofole had given her. She took some leaves to Accra to consult a botanist. He was helpful, but there were still gaps in her knowledge. She returned to Kumasi, determined to cultivate Ofole further.

After that she went for walks with her witch doctor friend to try to collect the specimens fresh so that they would be more easily identifiable. She made friends with other witch doctors too. Gradually she acquired a collection unique both in material and in knowledge. She could now cure the dread diseases herself, provided that she prepared the specimens in the African witch manner. She felt that this would not be practicable in Britain. She felt that the time had come for a big pharmaceutical firm to take an interest. She was convinced that here was a sedative that was better than any known drug which relaxed spasm without paralysing.

She went over the procedure many times in her mind. The findings of the active principles of the treatment and how they worked; the transfer to the laboratory and eventually to the wards of European hospitals where at least something could be done to help the unfortunate people who developed these fatal diseases. Her observations on *kwashiorkor* might affect Africa profoundly, but her observations on tetanus and meningitis might tame some of the most terrifying diseases known in Europe.

In great excitement she eventually went to England on leave.

She went straight to a big pharmaceutical firm, and said that she needed a good analytical chemist who would come to the Gold Coast and find out what the active principles in this treatment were. But the firm wasn't interested. Slowly the truth dawned on Cicely. In Britain tetanus, though serious and often fatal, was not common enough to make it profitable to find a cure. Moreover, scientists were reluctant to believe that something new might come out of Africa.

She kept the witch doctor's preparations and had other plans for them when she was transferred later to Malaya. But they were all lost during the occupation of Singapore.

She always felt safe in Africa, moving about freely and often alone through the streets and visiting the houses. She was impressed at how little violence and theft there was. But occasionally she came across unpleasant characters, and there were a few burglars and confidence tricksters. Her first encounter with one of them was soon after she arrived in Accra. As she was moving into her bungalow, her belongings were being unloaded from a lorry. A man seemed to be helpful and she asked him who he was.

"I be for your gardener." This was the local way of saying that this was his job. Cicely took it for granted that he had been attached to her household by the Department of Health, because this was how the garden work was usually arranged. Occasionally she saw him cutting the grass and tidying up. But after a couple of weeks police came to her clinic, dragging him. They produced an order book from one of the commercial firms showing that various goods had been ordered, including two dozen tins of sardines, several dozen reels of cotton and a sewing machine. Each had been signed "Dr Williams". It was a firm from which Cicely had never ordered anything.

He went to prison for six months. When he came out he returned, smiling, and tried to install himself again in Cicely's house. But when she told him to go away and threatened to call the police, he went without making a scene or apparently bearing a grudge.

An incident occurred in Kumasi which upset her seriously. It began with a series of small losses from her bungalow. Money disappeared from her purse, earrings from her dressing table. There were about fifteen small losses at frequent intervals. Cicely sacked three or four good houseboys because she felt that they were the only people who were coming in and out of the bungalow and would be able to take these things so regularly. But the thefts continued. After a couple of months she became worried and went to the police. As a result men from the Department of Public Works put up a metal fixture over the windows, but it was useless because they only fixed it up on one side. It was easy to put one's hand inside the expanded metal and open the other half of the window.

One night there were celebrations for the Jubilee of King George V, but Cicely was in bed with fever. Feeling ill, and half-dozing in the bedroom, she heard a small scratching noise. Her first reaction was a feeling that there was something nasty about such as a cockroach. She opened her eyes and saw a dark silent figure leaning over the table beside her bed. She was deeply afraid but also inquisitive, and wanted to see who it was. Automatically she called out, "Who's there? What is it?" Instantly the man leapt at her. Luckily for her she had a new strong mosquito net, and enough presence of mind to swing round and kick. She switched on the light over her bed and he ran into the dressing-room. She pursued him, but he picked up a chair and came at her with it. She saw that he was an Ashanti man with his hair cut in a peculiar way. He was greased all over and was wearing a pair of khaki shorts with pockets sewn on in black thread.

She ran to the front door, opened it and screamed loudly. The women's bungalows had been put among the men's with the idea that if there was trouble the women could scream for help. But her neighbour on one side was in Accra celebrating the Jubilee, and the other neighbour was in hospital with jaundice. She screamed louder, and the man jumped at her again. This time the houseboys living in the compound at the back of the house woke and ran to her rescue. The burglar fled.

Her friends were very kind and offered her guns and dogs and all sorts of things to keep her safe. The police were also kind and she accepted a police whistle, and for the next year slept with it tied round her neck, clutched in her right hand. During the whole of that year she found it difficult to sleep at all. Night after night she was awake waiting for the next burglar to come.

The police arrested some men and there were several identification parades, but Cicely never saw her assailant again. She became increasingly jittery and exhausted, and this was made worse by frequent night calls to the hospital. The police continued to search for the burglar, and said that they would give her a guard at night for the bungalow. She found this comforting, though she often knew that he was there only because of the snores. He seemed unable to stay awake, but she hoped the noise he made while asleep would frighten the burglars away.

In the summer of that year, 1936, her nervous state was improved by a visitor. He was Dr Cunningham Brown from the Colonial Office, and had come to Africa to look at mental hospitals. He was a lively man of independent mind, who interpreted his orders widely and argued that in order to understand what was going on in a mental hospital you had to understand what was going on in the community that it served. He realised that Cicely was steeped in African customs and ways of life, and he was keen to listen to her for as long as she would talk.

"Many people mock the Government child health work," she told him. "They say that there's already a land hunger, and that if these children are sick they had better die, for what's the point of looking after them? But I believe that these attitudes are wrong. This country is underpopulated, and there's room for millions more people in the Gold Coast. Besides, Africans are immensely responsive to education and easily acquire a sense of responsibility. Our business is to improve the quality of the population then the quantity can take care of itself."

"What is your impression of the attitude of the Europeans to the Africans?"

"I think that all of us who work closely with Africans respect them for their ability to learn what they wish to learn. Difficulty sometimes arises because their conventions about honesty are different from ours. Their first job is to look after their families, and many of them only get an education at all because an uncle or another member of the family has falsified some accounts or stolen something. I would say that in many cases you find that anything is regarded as justified as long as it is for the benefit of your own family."

"Yes. It's probably a stage in development. After all, it's only when people begin to get broader ideas of loyalties that they feel that honesty must be observed towards those outside their immediate family. What else?"

"Another difficulty is that many people who come out here have been brought up entirely in England and have never talked to coloured people in their lives. They find it hard to envisage that negroes can be educated and become judges and doctors. I think they are also often embarrassed about this. It isn't really a question of race antagonism. It's often awkwardness due to shyness in people who have never before had the benefit of working with other races. They are embarrassed simply by the new experience of talking to someone who happens to have a black face."

He was particularly interested in her adventures with the African witch doctors. It was his impression that they also treated much mental disease.

Cicely agreed. "Oh yes, indeed. There's a good deal of hysteria out here, but the Africans seem to take it in their stride. They often say 'this no be white man's sickness' and it's dealt with by the local people, often by witch doctors using some sort of sedatives. I have seen them measure out a handful or two of herbs which knock the patient out for a day or two. And they often come round in quite a different frame of mind."

Later it occurred to Cicely that this was rather like the "deep narcosis" treatment used in Western psychiatry.

"Very much the sort of thing," Brown commented, "I met while I was looking at mental hospitals in Nigeria. Once I went to a district up-country and said to the District Commissioner, 'Do you have many mental cases who have to be sent to hospital here?' He said, 'Certainly not.' So I went to the local chief and asked, 'Do you have many mental cases among your people?' And he said, 'Oh yes, very many'. So I asked him what he did with them. 'Oh,' said the chief, 'we send them to our local doctors and they seem to manage them very well." So I made a point of going with my interpreter to the compound of one of the local witch doctors, who agreed most pleasantly to my seeing his patients. We sat down and interviewed a whole row of them. One of them was a typical African woman. Her hair was stiff and on end and she wore nothing about the waist but a string of beads. I asked her some questions through the interpreter, but then I noticed that her answers were coming before the question had been translated. So I said, 'I think you understand English.' 'Oh, yes,' she said, 'perfectly.' 'Where did you learn it?' I asked, and, believe it or not, she answered, 'At the London School of Economics'."

They both laughed. Then he asked her more about her work, and she told him of the study she had been making of child health in the Gold Coast.

"I'm impressed with your diligence," he said. "What exactly are you doing it for? After all, I'm paid specifically to come here and do my survey. You seem to be doing yours just for fun, or at least out of a high sense of duty."

"And the glory of a gown."

"I beg your pardon?"

"The gown of a Doctor of Medicine at Oxford is crimson with scarlet silk sleeves and collar, and you wear it with a flat, round, black doctor's hat. It was my father's ambition that I should become a true and proper doctor. Most of us are only called 'doctor' by courtesy, you know. I want to have the right to wear it. It's beautiful."

She threw her head back as though already walking up the aisle towards the Vice-Chancellor, and there was a faint pink on her usually pale cheeks.

Towards the end of the year she left Kumasi and went on leave. Her thesis on Child Health in the Gold Coast was accepted without question by the University. She went up to Oxford to receive her degree, escorted by her uncle and cousin. The Sheldonian was being repaired, and the ceremony took place in the Divinity School under the Gothic fan vaulting where Rowland Williams had so often sat in his youth. Cicely remembered his describing it to her. She was pleased and proud that at last she was entitled to wear this gorgeous apparel.

She was due to return to the Gold Coast in December, but a few days before her departure she received a letter from the Colonial Office to say that she was to be transferred to Malaya. This was a shock. She had many regrets in not going back to Africa, not least because most of her possessions were still there. But within a couple of days she felt more cheerful, and she wrote to her mother, "On the whole it's probably a good thing. As a woman Medical Officer I can never get promotion. They have never given a higher post to a woman. If I can't move perpendicularly in the Service I may as well move horizontally."

A few days later she boarded a P. & O. liner for Singapore.

CHAPTER V

"HOW GREEN IT is," said Cicely, trying to appreciate the forests and rubber plantations. In Singapore island she was feeling homesick for hot, brown Africa.

"It's like that all over Malaya," said her cousin John. He was in the Army and lived with his wife at Changi on the eastern tip of the island. Cicely had been pleased to accept their invitation to stay until she found a bungalow or flat near the hospital. Today he was driving her into Singapore to be introduced to her new job at the General Hospital.

"Not so long ago the whole island was a snake-infested swamp. Raffles must have been a genius to recognise its possibilities." He pointed out the hill of Bukit Timah, the highest on the island. "It looks very British now." They drove along the coast towards the city, with its fine Government buildings and large European shops and offices. "It looks like any British possession. Houses, shops, hotels, churches, wide streets and hundreds of motor cars. But take a closer look at the people."

"They all seem to be Chinese."

"Most of them are. The Chinese also own most of the shops. If you look down those narrow, crowded lanes you can imagine that you're in China."

"What's that policeman?"

"He's a Malay. So is that van-driver."

"Aren't the Malays in rather a privileged position?"

"Indeed, yes. But after all it is their country. The British Government looks on everyone else as temporary foreigners. Malaya is said to have a government of the Chinese by the British for the Malays. But I don't think you'll find much racial discrimination in the Health Service. It's more marked in education, which is free for Malays but not for the others."

"Who are those women?"

"They aren't women, though visitors often think they are. They are Malay men wearing the national skirt or sarong practically down to their feet, with a feminine blouse called a 'baju' draped loosely over it. You don't see many Malay women because they aren't usually allowed out in the streets."

"There don't seem to be many women of any kind."

"That's one of the features of Singapore and one of its problems. It's a predominantly male city. Thousands of Chinese come to work here and don't bring their families, and there are also many workers from other parts of the Far East and Europe. As a result there's a great deal of prostitution and trafficking in opium."

"There seem to be a number of Indians too."

"Yes. Look, there's one draped in white. He is one of the 'chetties' or moneylenders. Many of the policemen are Sikhs or Punjabis, and so are the watchmen you see at night sleeping on truckle beds outside the stores and offices. There are also many Tamils working mostly as clerks or as manual workers, mending roads or driving bullock carts. Even in this fairly fashionable part of the town you can see the occasional Tamil walking along dressed only in a loin-cloth. And that man standing outside his shop wearing a fez like an Egyptian is an Iraqi from Baghdad."

"It's all so different from Africa. I find it confusing."

At the hospital she was met by a polite Indian doctor. He told her that he had trained at the King Edward VII College of medicine in Singapore and had worked for two years in England. He then explained her job to her. She was to work in the Women's Out-patients, where Malay was spoken by most people. He explained to her that there were Chinese amahs who could speak Malay and would interpret to the Chinese patients.

"But I don't speak Malay."

This possibility had not occurred to him. After a little thought and much conferring with his colleagues, he put her in charge of two wards containing about fifty women in each and asked her please to learn Malay as quickly as possible.

She found this language easy, and learnt more in a few weeks than she had learnt of any West African language in years. Because Malay was a *lingua franca* people acknowledged differences in pronunciation and understood that different foreigners speak it in different ways. If one tried to speak a West African language in Ghana one had to be pretty accurate before anybody would make an effort to understand. But in Singapore everyone made some effort to interpret what she was trying to say. But she was still homesick for Africa. She missed its initiative and ebullience. Everything in the Far East seemed so quiet and reserved.

The pattern of disease was very different from what she had seen in Africa. The women's wards were full of chronic cases of beri-beri, and there were also a number of women who had tried to commit suicide. If a Chinese woman was upset, the popular way to commit suicide was to drink caustic soda. But often they did not die at once. They were in hospital for many months with obstruction due to scarring of the gullet, in considerable pain, and slowly starving to death because they couldn't swallow.

With so many long-term cases Cicely thought that these women should not merely lie in bed and think about their miseries, but should move about as soon as they were able and help each other, bringing glasses of water, mending sheets, washing towels and doing any little job that could be found for them. But she ran into trouble from the nursing authorities because Matron didn't like the mess.

A serious epidemic of typhoid came to Singapore. It was finally traced to a man who made ice-cream in a lavatory pail and sold it to schoolchildren. During this epidemic most patients were too ill to move about. One day the Matron came into the ward and spoke to Cicely brightly.

"I like the typhoid epidemic because your wards look so tidy."

"It is tidier still in the mortuary," snorted Cicely. When angry she had a quick tongue.

She also had to watch carefully for exploitation of patients. Occasionally she would find an amah charging 5 cents for a glass of water or 10 cents for a bedpan. This also she had never experienced in Africa.

One of her duties was to look after women who had been brought in by the police or who were under observation, either as prisoners or to be signed up and sent to a mental hospital. She discovered that her predecessor had usually signed these forms without questioning them, but Cicely was often not satisfied and insisted on going into the case. This was difficult because she could only do it through a Chinese nurse whose English was likely to be limited. It was difficult to persuade the nurses to be patient and to translate accurately enough for her to make a personal assessment.

One day a woman was brought in by the police because she had jumped into Singapore Harbour. A nurse agreed to translate but took a more active part than Cicely wished.

"Of course, doctor, she is mad. She threw herself into the harbour. Of course she is mad."

"Never mind that. Let's see why she did it."

"She tried to drown herself in the harbour. She is mad."

Cicely tried to begin at the beginning. "Ask her why she jumped into the harbour."

There was a swift interchange between the nurse and the patient.

"Doctor, she said it was because her little girl went to tea with her uncle. You see, that just shows you. Of course she is mad, flinging herself into the harbour for such a reason."

Cicely went back to the beginning yet once more and gradually the whole story came out. The woman's husband had been working in Singapore, but had suddenly died of pneumonia. She had no close relatives in the village in China where she was living, but a well-to-do uncle of her husband who lived in Singapore wrote and suggested that she should come with her little girl to live in his household, where the child would be educated. On the ship she became friendly with some other Chinese, who said that they lived in Singapore and knew the uncle. They had a little boy two years older than the girl. They said that perhaps one day they would arrange a marriage between the little girl and the little boy. When they arrived in Singapore Harbour the two families were together at the Customs and the woman was talking to an official about the luggage. She looked round and saw the other family speeding off in a rickshaw with her child, and that was the last she had seen of her. For three days she had been wandering round Singapore in great distress, and her situation was complicated by the fact that she spoke an unusual form of Chinese. She had been unable to find the family or the uncle or the little girl, and she had eaten and drunk nothing since she arrived. In the end she had jumped into the harbour.

Cicely had been in Singapore for about six months when the doctor in charge of the children's wards was promoted to an administrative post. This gave her a chance to look after the children's wards, which was what she really wanted to do. She also now had a bungalow near the hospital in Orange Grove Road, which was two miles from the hospital but much nearer than Changi. While she was living with her cousins she had always been uneasy about being so far from her patients. Now she could keep a closer watch on them and do a night round.

But when her cousins came to dinner she was so distressed about the conditions in the children's wards that she found it difficult to be sociable.

"I have 120 beds for children," she told them, "and the mortality rate is dreadful. We admit so many children dying of beri-beri that we had to make a special hospital bye-law for children who die in the lift on their way to the wards! When you remember that beri-beri, like most of the other diseases they have, is preventable, it makes you want to cry. It's all so unnecessary."

"Why does it happen?"

"As things are at present I have no out-patients and no opportunity to see my patients before their diseases are too far advanced for cure. There's no opportunity to treat the diseases in the early stages when it is usually possible to prevent a catastrophe. It's largely a question of the relationship between us and the Municipal Council. Putting it bluntly, we don't get on well with them. Unfortunately, in the town of Singapore all the child welfare work is done through the Municipality and not through the Government. They have good welfare centres for infants but they don't even bother about children after they're a year old, and so we usually don't see them until they're dying. I'm trying to start an out-patients clinic associated with the wards, but I usually have to look after 120 beds without even a house physician to help me, so I don't have much time to do clinics as well."

Dinner was served on the verandah by Ali, Cicely's excellent Malay houseboy.

"Pork?" John looked at Ali in some surprise. Most Malays are Moslems.

"He's obliging," said Cicely. "He doesn't mind cooking pork as long as he has a long fork."

"He seems to be a treasure."

"He is. He's clean and quick and quiet. The child you saw when you arrived is Mina, his wife. She's only about fifteen. She is supposed to help in the house too, but if I ask her to do anything she collapses in giggles on the bed. But Ali does everything so well that it doesn't matter."

"What about the nursing at the hospital?" asked one of her cousins, realising that Cicely really wanted to talk about her work.

"It's very different from what I was used to in West Africa, and I think this makes the situation with the children even more difficult. The hospital is a big training school for nurses, and they come to the children's wards for only two months, just to get some experience with children. There's little continuity of care for the patients. Many of the nurses seem to look on a baby in the cot as just something that has to have a feed at one end and a napkin at the other. They have no interest in the children as people and no possibility of learning about their backgrounds. It's very frustrating. And another difficulty is that the nurses hate to come into my wards because all we have is an endless succession of dying babies."

"Isn't there a chance to admit the mothers too? You used to do that in West Africa, didn't you?"

"I have room for about ten which I suppose is better than nothing. But in the Gold Coast every child was always accompanied by the mother or an elder sister or somebody associated with it. I think it makes a tremendous difference."

Mina, the fifteen-year-old wife of Cicely's houseboy Ali, was pregnant, and her small, scarcely adult body was swelling under her sarong. She was always gay and wore tinkling anklets and flowers in her hair. But Cicely was worried.

"You must eat good food, Mina," she said, making sure that Ali could hear. "It is important for the health of your baby. You must have eggs and tomatoes and under-milled rice." This was the sort of diet she always recomended to Malays.

But Mina just giggled and adjusted the flowers in her hair.

"She will return to her father's house in the town for the birth of the baby," said Ali. "It is the Malay custom." He liked to do things as they should be done. He bowed politely and handed Cicely a newly-delivered letter. While she was opening it the door-bell rang, and he went off to answer it.

The letter was from the Rotary Club asking her to speak to them. "How can I do that?" she thought. "I only know about babies. I can't talk about anything else. But if I announce that I'm going to talk about babies nobody will come. No one really cares about babies."

Ali returned with Wong Lok-Kwan, Cicely's senior health nurse. Cicely sometimes gave her a lift to the hospital in her car. The houseboy returned to the kitchen, and through the half-opened door Cicely caught a glimpse of Mina tucking into a bowl of white rice.

She drove most of the way to the hospital without speaking, busy with her thoughts about Mina's pregnancy, about problems in the children's wards and about her forthcoming talk to the Rotary Club. Wong Lok-Kwan sat demurely beside her.

"The food habits in this country are terrible," said Cicely at last.

"You mean people like him, Doctor?" asked Wong Lok-Kwan, indicating an old man at a street corner. He was offering bits of cabbage, probably picked out of dustbins, at one cent a handful.

"Partly."

"There's not as much real poverty as you might think. We Chinese have our *kongsi*."

"The secret and subversive societies?"

"That's not true. They are really a system of helping each other. You pay your dues to your *kongsi* and that assures you of shelter and a certain amount to eat. When you get work you pay more to the leaders of your *kongsi*. Of course it does lead to some disgraceful things happening. But these societies are usually formed for protection and certainly, as a result, most people have enough to eat."

"I was thinking how little natural sense we humans have about what to eat. Most of the diseases we see here are due to people choosing the wrong food."

"Is it not the same in England?"

"In England most people eat better than here."

At the door of the ward was a Chinese woman with a baby. It was thin and wrinkled, weak and hungry.

"I have brought you this baby, Miss Doctor, because his mother is dead and there is no food for him."

"Why don't you feed the baby with milk from a bottle?"

"We have no money to buy the bottle."

"Can you buy the milk?"

"We have no money at all."

"When did the mother die?"

"Last Thursday, Doctor."

"How much did it cost to bury the mother?"

The woman smiled proudly. "We paid 210 Malay dollars."

"210 dollars!" repeated Cicely, angrily. "Twenty-six pounds sterling and not one sixpence left to buy milk for the baby!" She turned to her nurse. "Do you have to observe the conventions no matter what the cost?"

Wong Lok-Kwan looked at her feet.

"I suppose it is a question of face," she said.

"Even if the family starve?"

"It's true."

"Faith and customs! Customs and faith! No wonder the babies die. Look at the prestige value you attach to your food. You seem to think that food is good just because it comes from China. All those salted vegetables! They have no goodness in them."

She turned to the student nurses.

"These wards are full of beri-beri, which is due to deficiency of vitamin B1 and is usually caused by eating polished rice. It is a dreadful thing for your people. For if you would only eat the under-milled rice which you now give to the chickens, your people would not get this beri-beri and your children would not die. It's not a question of money. In the side ward down the corridor there is a little Chinese boy who is dying of the disease. His father is a millionaire."

"Why is there so little beri-beri among the Indians, Doctor?" asked a quiet girl in a sari.

"Because their customs are different. They eat rice which has been steamed under pressure, and this drives the vitamin B1 into the centre of the grain so that even if the outside is removed you can't get beri-beri if you eat it."

"But Indian rice tastes funny," said a Chinese student with a giggle. There were murmurs of agreement down the line.

"Yes," said Cicely with passion. "It tastes funny to you because you're not used to it. If you were sensible you would start getting used to it now so that you can teach your patients from personal experience, and when you marry and have children of your own they will be in no danger from beri-beri."

An understanding smile passed between her and the student. Cicely was pleased. Most of the medical students and nurses were ignorant and prejudiced but wonderfully open to teaching.

"Now, Sister, what is that baby in the corner?"

"He has just come in, Doctor. He is nine days old. His mother died in childbirth."

"Just look at his eyes! They're practically destroyed!"

Gently, Cicely bent over the tiny, wizened creature. He

whimpered and twitched. She examined him all over, peering, patting, tapping, listening. The group waited politely round the cot. At last Cicely looked up.

"Keratomalacia. I've never seen it in so young a child." She turned to one of the nurses. "How has this baby been fed?"

"I don't know, Doctor."

"Then I'll make a guess. I think almost certainly it has been fed from birth with sweetened condensed milk."

"Quite right," said Sister. "I asked the grandmother who brought the baby in."

"Just as I thought. He will be blind for the rest of his life because he was fed on tinned milk!"

"But in the newspapers, Doctor, it says that sweetened condensed milk is the right food for babies."

"Don't believe advertisements, nurse. Unscrupulous milk firms are conducting a wicked campaign to persuade mothers to give up breast feeding and to feed their babies with sweetened condensed milk."

"They send round people they call 'nurses'."

"All the worse," said Cicely. "They are doing terrible things to the children."

"But, Doctor," piped a little Chinese girl who had so far kept in the background, "surely it is unseemly to encourage the growth of the breasts. A Chinese girl is taught by her mother to bind her breasts very tightly. We don't want to feed our babies like animals. Every Chinese woman of good family wears a tight bodice."

"And probably deforms her breasts so that she can't feed her baby, even if it's a matter of life and death. Your customs are killing your children, nurse, for as things are in Singapore today, artificial feeding is dangerous for babies. Look for yourselves." She pointed at the blind baby. "You can see that what I say is true."

She paused in her outburst and was pleased to see that the students looked impressed. She felt convinced that they were taking in what she said, and she continued:

"You must do what you can to counteract the work of these

milk firms. You nurses are the proper people to do it, for you belong here, you know the people, and yet you have been well trained and have the opportunity to know what is true and right. You can do much to teach the mothers the proper way to care for their babies. And, my God, it is needed!" She turned back to the baby. "Give it the special drops with every feed, please, Sister."

She passed on to the next bed.

"That child looks very pale. Has he had convulsions? Yes, just as I thought. Lead poisoning! And you can see the white powder still on his face. Look at that blood report. The baby is dying because Chinese people admire a fair complexion. Your custom of rubbing lead powder into your children's faces to preserve a fair skin is even more dangerous than feeding the child with tinned milk."

"But what else can one do, Doctor?" asked one of the students. "Only coolies and workmen get sunburnt."

"You must change your ideas and those of your people. It is the only way. We in England have changed and are changing all the time. At one time it was fashionable to be as pale as possible, and no one who was anyone went out into the sun, just as it is now here. But with us the fashion has changed. We know that the sun, in moderate doses, is a good thing, and nowadays white people like to look a little brown. Look at this baby and see the terrible things that can happen through trying to make the skin whiter."

She wrote on the treatment chart at the foot of the bed.

"A woman with a baby is waiting to see you, Doctor."

The woman was a poor Chinese. She was undernourished, poorly dressed, and looked as though she expected someone to hit her. She spoke only Chinese, and Cicely had to use one of the nurses as an interpreter. She examined the baby and spoke to the nurse.

"Tell the mother that the baby has something wrong inside and must come into hospital. It is also important for the baby to be breast fed. Tell her we can give her a bed near the baby so that she can feed him."

The nurse translated. Immediately the woman became agitated. Tears spilt out of her eyes as she talked rapidly. Eventually the nurse turned to Cicely and said:

"She says she cannot stay in hospital because if she does not go home at once her husband will sell the two other children. He is a gambler and always needs money. He has already sold one child. It happened one day when she was out looking for cabbage stalks in dustbins because she had no food for her family."

"If that is the situation," said Cicely, "she had better go home at once, for even if she stays she will probably lose her milk from worry."

The woman dumped the baby into Cicely's arms with a thankful look and hurried away.

"This buying and selling of children is terrible," said Cicely. "How much would this baby be worth on the open market?"

"Sick like that, perhaps 2 or 3 dollars."

"And her children at home?"

"A healthy little boy may fetch 200 to 300 Malay dollars."

"£35," muttered Cicely to herself. Aloud she said, "I'm afraid that the difference is the profit we often make for the touts. They go to a mother and say 'Your baby doesn't look very well. I'll give you 2 dollars for it.' Then they bring the baby to the hospital. If it recovers they can sell it again as a healthy child."

"Talking about touts," said Sister, "that woman who often brings in babies called about the little girl she brought in last week. She was most indignant when I told her that the child was dead, and said, 'There now, I've lost all that stuff I gave for it'."

"What did she give for it?"

"She paid 2 dollars, a kati of mee,* six eggs and six pigs' trotters."

Afterwards in the corridor Wong Lok-Kwan said, "You know, Doctor Williams, the children who are bought and sold in this way are not always badly treated. Many are better off than before. The wife of an important Malay official comes to

* 2lb. of noodles.

Singapore every year to buy little Chinese girls. She takes the children back and brings them up in her household."

"I know the one you mean. I've seen her. It is curious to see those girls with Chinese features but with Malay attitudes and manners. What happens to them when they grow up?"

"She marries them off as wives or concubines to her sons or to other members of her family."

"I suppose she feels that they whiten up the Malayan complexion?"

"That is true," said Wong Lok-Kwan. "She is, of course, also bringing souls to Islam, so that buying Chinese girls is a means of acquiring merit."

"All the same," said Cicely, "this trafficking in children is evil. I should like to start a place where we could supervise adoptions and where children could be taken in who need care and protection. People who wish to adopt children could come and get them, and we should have some check on where they went. As things are at the moment, many people with little money and more children than they want solve the problem by giving a child to a richer relative or selling it to someone who can afford more children. I have seen many cases where children were sold for immoral purposes."

"My husband is a policeman," said Wong Lok-Kwan. "He says that the Government Department does try to protect girls."

"That is true, but I am sure that he knows, even better than I do, what goes on. On the way home we will go to the Salvation Army Hostel where I can show you how tragedy can arise, even with the best will in the world."

She told the nurse about a child called Peter.

Cicely had a good working relationship with the Salvation Army, who ran a home for mothers and children. They would take in a mother and child or a child on its own from Cicely's wards, and she found this very useful. In return she visited their children and gave medical advice whenever they asked for it. One of Cicely's favourites was a child who had been born literally in the gutter. The mother died and the child was taken into the Home. He was about eighteen months old. They called him Peter and he did not thrive, though nothing definite was wrong with him. One day an American lady who had been to Cicely's First Aid classes at the Y.M.C.A. came to see her in the hostel and asked, "What is wrong with that child?" Cicely answered, "What he needs is love." Later that day she happened to meet the woman's husband, and he said, "We'll take him, Doctor." At first Cicely did not understand. Then he said, "My wife tells me that you have a child in the hostel who needs love. We'll take him." So Peter was taken to their home and given a nursery. There were three Chinese women servants in the house, a Malay driver or syce and a Malay gardener. They were all summoned and shown Peter's weight chart pinned on the wall. They were told that if the weight went up, they would all get an increase in pay. If the weight went down it would be reduced. Peter enjoyed himself. He began to smile and to gain weight. But unfortunately an emergency arose and the Americans had to leave Singapore. They seriously considered adopting the child but in the end they decided that it would be unwise, at that time, to take a Chinese child back to America as their adopted son. So poor Peter was returned to the Hostel.

They found him sitting in the corner, a lost soul, rocking his head from side to side and making a growling, inhuman noise.

"He hasn't eaten since he came back," said the Salvation Army major.

"He'll die if we don't find another home for him," said Cicely. "He isn't the sort of child who can cope with an institution."

"I have hopes," said the Salvation Army lady. "We have heard of some rich Chinese who wish to adopt a son."

"The sooner the better," said Cicely. "By the time another few days have passed I think anyone who sees him will be scared to take him."

"I'll drive back through the Chinese quarters," said Cicely. "I want to visit a baby."

"Which baby, Doctor?"

"One of those with early keratomalacia due to sweetened

condensed milk. I was particularly interested because the mother, unlike so many of the Chinese women, has plenty of milk and is willing to feed the baby herself. But she's weak-willed and submits to any pressures that come her way. She didn't turn up at the hospital this afternoon, though I specially asked her to come."

She parked her car and they walked down a narrow alley full of Chinese shops and overhung with gay Chinese signs. At the end was a big building, four storeys high. Cicely and Wong Lok-Kwan began to climb the swaying wooden staircase. The building was arranged in the typical manner of poor Chinese houses, with each floor divided into eight or nine cubicles not more than about 8 feet square. Each cubicle housed a whole family, many with five or six children. Only the cubicles at each end of the row had windows. The only kitchen in the building, for perhaps thirty families or more, was in the basement, which also housed the only tap and lavatory. These appalling quarters were made worse by the Chinese tendency to collect everything they could. In contrast to the Malays, whom Cicely usually found neat and tidy in their quarters and very clean, the Chinese cubicles were often filled with bits of silver paper, cigarette packets and all sorts of scraps that they had collected like magpies.

They found the woman at the top of the building in a cubicle without a window. It contained even more litter than most cubicles. The baby hung in a sarong, suspended from the roof by a string. It looked ill and swollen. Several small children were sitting on the floor chewing. At the sight of the two women the mother jumped guiltily.

"The baby is ill again. You haven't been doing what I said," said Cicely, sternly.

The woman looked at her feet.

"Why not?" Cicely's voice was now friendly and encouraging.

"The lady came and told me not to give the breast."

"What lady?"

"The nurse lady. She bring milk in tin and say it better for baby. She say it not good to feed baby like you say. Breasts not good, not nice. Like animals."

"My God," said Cicely to Wong Lok-Kwan. "The milk firms! They are undermining everything that we do. They're killing off the children wholesale. What a terrible state of affairs."

She sat down on a low stool, and spoke slowly and serious to the mother.

"Now, I want you to listen very carefully. The lady who came to see you was not a nurse. She was a saleslady who wants you to spend your money on tins of milk for your baby. But her milk is not good for your baby. You can see for yourself that the baby is sick again. The lady doesn't care about your baby. She only wants you to buy the tins so that she can get the money for them. Do you understand? Everything the lady said to you was because she wants your money. If you do what she says your baby will be sick."

The woman nodded miserably. Slowly and patiently Cicely repeated the instructions she had given her in the hospital a week before. When she had finished the woman took down her baby from the sarong and gave him her breast. Cicely could see that she had plenty of milk, and after delivering a final exhortation she left.

"I suppose she'll be all right till next time," she said bitterly to Wong Lok-Kwan as they went down the stairs.

"You're right about her being weak," said the Chinese woman. "If the woman from the milk firm comes again she'll go back on to the tin."

"Yes," said Cicely, vehemently. "These wicked profiteers are dragging healthy lactating breasts out of babies' mouths and pouring in their beastly patent milks. The situation is getting out of hand."

They emerged into the street, blinking their eyes after the semi-darkness of the Chinese house.

"These houses where the poor Chinese live are like beehives," said Cicely, taking a big breath of air. "The living conditions are fantastic."

She was silent most of the way home, seething with problems.

"I've got it," she said explosively, at last. "I'll start a war on these milk firms and try to instil some sense of responsibility into them. I'll start my campaign at the Rotary Club. I'll call my talk 'Milk and Murder', for that's what it amounts to."

A few weeks later she and Wong Lok-Kwan went out with one of her most able Health Sisters, Kathleen Mackintosh, and her policeman husband, who in later years became a distinguished Commissioner of Police in Hong Kong. They dressed in trousers and carried guns. He took them to opium dens and houses of prostitution. They saw down-and-outs living in the rubbish pits and shelters made from bits of newspaper and cardboard and tin cans. They saw dead babies lying on rubbish dumps where they had been thrown. She had never seen such appalling conditions, but could not fail to admire the courage and dignity with which human beings faced them.

"The town is expanding rapidly," said Duncan Mackintosh. "It's impossible for the social services to keep pace with the changes. But the object of police work is not just to punish crime but to discover how crime can be prevented. This is a tremendous job and needs a lot of co-operation between your department, mine, and the Education department."

CHAPTER VI

ALI RETURNED SMILING from his father-in-law's house and said to Cicely, "It's a boy, a beautiful boy."

Through his joy Cicely could sense a small feeling of triumph at her expense. Lately there had been tension between them. Cicely had shown much concern over Mina during her pregnancy, and had repeatedly encouraged her to change her habits, particularly her diet. But Mina had taken no notice. In giving birth to a beautiful boy she seemed to have justified herself.

Cicely was delighted and said so. Ali cleaned and polished the bungalow even more cheerfully than usual. He was anxious for Cicely to come to his father-in-law's house to see the baby, and this she eagerly agreed to do. But two days later, on the morning of her proposed visit, he was in tears.

"The baby is dead, Doctor. He died suddenly in the night."

Cicely was certain that the baby had died of beri-beri due to Mina's inadequate diet. She felt that Mina's behaviour during her pregnancy and her attitude to it had been typically Malay. In contrast to the Africans, Chinese and Indians, Cicely usually found the Malays carefree and feckless. They looked upon it as a matter of fate whether or not their children survived. She would often say to a Malay mother, "What has happened to the baby?" "Oh, it has died." And she would say "What a pity." And the reply would be, "What the Lord Allah wishes." Cicely would say vehemently, "But the Lord Allah doesn't wish it at all. He gave you a beautiful baby. It died because you are careless. The Lord Allah wants you to use your brain and look after the baby properly." But it was difficult to persuade the Malays to show responsibility in the way she wished. Even though they had advantages of education and special privileges in housing, their infant mortality was much higher than that of the Chinese and the Indians. Cicely felt that this was partly due to their religion. They were Moslems, and for them divorce was easy. The husband had only to say three times to his wife "Tolak, tolak, tolak", and she was divorced. This insecurity often had a disastrous effect on the mentality of the women. They felt that they must make the most of their youth and beauty while it lasted, and some of them exchanged their husbands in rapid succession, knowing that once they were old and less desirable it would be more difficult to get a man to protect them or to provide for them.

The Chinese attitude was different again and also a shock to Cicely, accustomed as she was to the devotion of the Africans, who showed their love of their children in ways which were easy for a European to appreciate and admire. The Chinese were more difficult to understand. Chinese mothers were fond of their children, but in many families economic necessity came first. As with the Africans, to have many children was a sign of wealth and therefore conferred prestige, but of a different sort. The Chinese in Malaya were an overpopulated community. It was grand if you could show that you had three wives, four concubines and twenty children. But if you had no money then you didn't have these status symbols and children were sacrificed to economic need. In the seven years that she had spent in Ghana, Cicely found only two abandoned children. In Singapore there were thousands.

From a doctor's point of view there were advantages in the Chinese attitude to children, and among these was the possibility of good pathological studies. It was easy to get permission to carry out post-mortem examinations, and they did a great number. Many Chinese regarded the hospital as a place where they could consign their dying children. They liked to make a funeral an occasion for ritual and display, but if they couldn't afford an impressive funeral they often preferred to have none. Most parents of children who died in hospital had no objection to a post-mortem if the hospital would provide for the burial of the child. Some people came to the hospital, dumped a dying baby and ran away without giving an address. It was a way of disposing of an unwanted corpse.

Thus Cicely learnt that the attitude towards children is something with a different flavour in each community.

When Mina became pregnant again Cicely said, "Any more dead babies and I'm going to sack both of you," and Mina smiled more seriously than before. This time she did what Cicely told her, ate the right food and took the right amount of exercise. The result was a beautiful boy. Ali and Mina were Cicely's devoted attendants and friends for ever, and little Fazil grew up fine and strong.

One day, to Cicely's delight, an old friend from West Africa turned up. George Young, having finished a tour of hospitals in Africa, had arrived in Singapore to do the same job in Malaya. They met for lunch. He seemed depressed.

"It's no good their sending me to the East," he said. "I'm saturated with Africa and it's hard to take in anything here."

"I know just how you feel. I felt like that myself after I arrived. Everything here seemed so vague and unimportant. I missed the vigour and vitality of Africa, and I felt as though I was swimming through cotton wool. At first I hated the people and the place and the work."

"And now?"

"It was a shock trying to pick up and to understand such a different social system. But I'm becoming fond of Singapore and I'm beginning to enjoy the life here. I'm getting to know the Chinese and to appreciate their extraordinary courage and hard work. I think they probably have the stiffest upper lips that God ever made. But I've come to value the real intelligence and astuteness of the Indians and the tremendous charm of the Malays."

"Tell me about life here."

She told him all that she had learnt: about the different attitudes to life and to children in the three main races, Chinese, Malay and Indian; of all the diseases that she saw in the hospital and outside; about the beri-beri and the problem of tinned milk.

"We even see rickets."

He looked incredulous. "Oh, surely not. Rickets is caused by lack of sunshine. I can't believe you can get it 3° north of the Equator."

"I thought that too. I could scarcely believe my eyes when I saw my first cases. But it's true. Many poor Chinese live in horrible little cubicles and never see the sun at all. Also people who live on rubber plantations may spend their whole lives under the heavy shade of the rubber trees in little dark huts. So we get quite a few cases from the rural areas as well as from the towns. Some of these babies have never been taken into the sun in their whole lives. Even if they are taken out the mothers cover them up. The Chinese admire a fair complexion, particularly in little girls."

"I think I ought to see some rubber plantations and something of the countryside in general before I really start looking at hospitals."

"Rubber is so much part of Malaya that it is difficult to remember that it isn't natural to it. I was astonished when I learnt that rubber trees were originally imported from Brazil to Kew Gardens and then taken to Malaya and cultivated. But I am driving up to Fraser's Hill tomorrow. Would you like to come?"

"What's Fraser's Hill?"

"It's a beautiful hill station about 250 miles up the West Coast of Malaya, beyond Kuala Lumpur. Doctors from the hospital here can go as medical officers for a couple of weeks whenever there's a vacancy. It's a wonderful change from the constant strain and sometimes very distressing work in the children's wards in Singapore. It has an excellent climate and is beautiful and green, with a golf course and exciting walks through the jungle."

"I'll come willingly. I want to visit people in that part of the country in any case. What's the social life like here in Singapore?"

"It suits me well on the whole. The European community here is much bigger than in Ghana. There are plenty of unmarried women so one isn't under the same pressure to be sociable. You can do more or less as you please. I particularly enjoy the swimming club. It's an old-fashioned club by the sea and you can always get a meal there. It's open all night and you can go there at any time, swim and then eat bacon and eggs, even at five o'clock in the morning."

"Isn't there some sort of celebration tonight?"

"Yes. For the Coronation. I'll take you."

Bright colours. Bright lights. Fireworks splashed across the sky. The dragon dancing round the beautiful decorated Chinese lanterns.

"I can't help feeling it's an awful waste of money," said the earnest young man.

"Yes," said Cicely remotely, drinking in all the colour and festivity. She was enjoying every firework and the bang of every gong and band. "If you think of all the terrible poverty perhaps it is rather bad to spend all this money on fireworks and decorations."

"I suppose people need opportunities for enjoyment, even if their tummies go empty," the young man replied doubtfully.

"It's a mistake to underrate the value of national celebrations. Look at that family in the street. Father, mother and four children all dressed up and holding hands. Look at their faces. Until I worked with the Chinese I never came across people who so much enjoyed dressing up and revelling in every spark of the fireworks. I think I appreciate it because I'm rather like that too."

Wistfully she thought of her beautiful scarlet doctor's gown in faraway Oxford.

"What's Tiger Balm?" asked George Young, "It's advertised all over the place."

They were driving across the causeway that carried road and railway across the narrow Straits of Johore. Huge hoardings spoilt the view of the glittering mountains on the mainland behind.

"It's a highly popular patent medicine, contents unknown.

They use it for anything from toothache to ingrowing toenails."

"So you take an interest in native medicine here too?"

"Yes, indeed, and I didn't have to look very far to find it. The Chinese *sinseh* or herbal doctors have an enormous trade, and I often stop in the market or in the shops to find out what they are selling."

"Found anything good?"

"Nothing as dramatic as the African treatment for tetanus and meningitis. But one of the big differences between the African local medicine and the Chinese is in the packaging, which the Chinese do beautifully. For instance, you can buy a snake's gall bladder in a dainty little white wax ball with beautiful red Chinese writing on the outside. Chinese medicines look so attractive that I'm not surprised people become addicted to them."

She told him about the Chinese hospital where patients were treated with Chinese indigenous medicine. She had made friends with the doctors there and sometimes visited it. She was interested to see how each patient was given a prescription which was then written on a piece of bamboo. The bamboo was taken to the dispensary, where the dispenser had drawers full of leaves and bits of root and powders, ground up crabs' eyes, locusts' legs and so on. He would take out the correct quantities of each and put them in a little glass pannikin. On the lid of the pannikin was placed the bamboo with the patient's name and the prescription. Outside the dispensary there was a row of little fires and all the pannikins were boiling. Thus each patient received his correct mixture.

"But sometimes children come to our hospital horribly cauterized. The Chinese do this with a joss stick heated in the fire and applied to any injured or septic part. There is also a good deal of skin disease among the Chinese because they don't wash sick children. The result is often appalling septic skin conditions. Some of the Chinese babies wear a garment called a *barat* which is a kind of bodice made out of stiff cloth with a rather stiff string round the neck. I've found that the *barat* often rubs the skin round the neck and starts septic sores."

"Why do you think there is such a lot of sepsis?"

"Partly because the children are kept indoors. The skin becomes white and flabby and seems to have no resistance. In the sun they improve. The babies in my ward are pushed out on to the balcony and the cautery marks heal."

"Do you ever send your own patients to be treated by native medicine?"

"No, but I once allowed a patient to be treated with it in my own hospital."

"How like you, Cicely. Do tell me about it."

"Well, you know that many children in my ward are suffering from neglect and from being left too much alone. We have one ward with seventy very ill children. Few mothers stay in hospital with them, and some children are orphans and have no one to visit them. Many are not getting on as they should. They don't get the individual attention that every child needs. One child was having all the medical treatment he needed but was not improving. I thought he was going to die. We had some excellent amahs who worked in the wards with the nurses, and one day I was looking at the child and a passing amah (a particularly good one whom we called Mrs Bottle) gave me a look, made a disparaging gesture and said to me, 'That baby has the monkey sickness.' I said, 'What is the monkey sickness?' She said, 'With the monkey sickness they look just like this.' So I said, 'Do you know any medicine which is good for the monkey sickness?' and she said, 'The sinseh round the corner has the medicine.' 'Would 2 dollars buy it?' I asked. She said, 'That would be plenty.' So I sent her to get it, and half an hour later she came back with some vines and powders and liquid and she said the most important thing is to tie these round the wrists and ankles and tummy. So we dolled up this poor little monkey-faced baby with vines and dried leaves, and of course word went round the hospital that Dr Williams was using native medicine in her ward and everyone came to see my monkey disease. The child promptly got well. Personally I think it was the result not of the vine leaves but of the extra attention."

"Fascinating," said George Young. "But I'm sorry you haven't found anything extraordinary like your cures for tetanus and meningitis."

He was gazing out of the window and changed the subject. "It's interesting how the mountain ranges are flanked by wide plains."

"Those plains are scarcely above sea level. When early explorers approached Malaya from the sea they saw the mountains sticking up at intervals and thought that the peninsula was a string of islands."

"And the mountains gleam so. I've never seen anything like it."

"That's quartz crystal and the origin of the Malay legend that the mountains are made of diamonds guarded by demons."

"This part of the jungle seems to be virtually uninhabited."

"Not as much as you might think. If you look closely you'll see a series of Malay villages with little thatched houses on stilts buried under the thick jungle growth of their gardens. You can drive through villages with thousands of inhabitants and scarcely notice them at all."

A colony of monkeys appeared, chattering as they swung from tree to tree. The treetops were covered with orchids and there were brightly coloured birds, butterflies at least 12 inches across from wing tip to wing tip, and huge, beautiful trees and tropical flowers.

"Do you have much to do with the countryside outside Singapore?"

"Increasingly so, largely because of my passion for linking preventive medicine with curative. I can't make any headway in Singapore itself. The municipality just doesn't want to know about it, and the result is that the hospital doctors aren't particularly interested in preventive medicine, or in the maintenance of health. But I believe that this attitude is wrong, and I've managed to establish good relations with the maternal and child health work that's being done, not in the Singapore municipality itself but in the rural areas round about. The rest of the island is run by the Government, and so this terrible split in administration doesn't occur."

Soon after she had taken over the children's wards Cicely had admitted a very sick child from a rural clinic. He turned out to have tuberculous meningitis, which in those days was always fatal. When he died Cicely returned the clinic card with the diagnosis written on it. Later, by chance, she discovered what happened as a result.

The card went back to the Matron in charge of all the rural centres, Miss I. N. M. Simmonds, a far-sighted and energetic Scotswoman. Miss Simmonds took action, which Cicely later learnt was typical of her. She went to the home of the child to try to find out if there was a possible source of tuberculosis there. She was convinced that no one in the child's family had tuberculosis. She did the same thing at the school. She then discovered that the child had been attending what they called a "Skola Arab", or Koran school where the teacher was an old man with a cough. She persuaded the old man to go to the local dispensary and tuberculosis was diagnosed. She then went to the Malay community in this village and explained that the man should not be teaching the children because he was a source of infection. She actually managed to persuade them to pension him off and to hire a new young Koran teacher.

Cicely was immensely impressed, and said to Wong Lok-Kwan, "That just shows you the sort of health work that can be done even under the difficult conditions out here. I must go and meet Miss Simmonds."

She discovered that the rural health clinics mostly started at 6 o'clock in the morning, the most convenient time for the rural people to attend. So one morning Cicely rose before dawn and drove out of Singapore.

In front of a small hut near a rubber plantation was a queue of perhaps 150 women with their children. It struck Cicely that they were all poor people in their party clothes. In this district they were almost certainly rubber tappers, yet no one wore working clothes.

Cicely was met by Miss Simmonds herself, a tiny, bird-like woman with a big mouth and smile. She had once been a Sister Tutor at Edinburgh.

"We cover nearly all the villages now," she told Cicely. "One after another the village headmen have come to me and said, 'We want you to start work in our village. We will build a house for the midwife. We will build a room where you can hold your clinics if you will give us a midwife.' In this way I have been able to expand my work."

"How tidy the patients look!"

"Yes, I believe that's important. Most of them live in poor conditions and have dirty work to do, but I expect them to be neat and clean at the clinic. I say to them, 'I have a bath before I come. I expect you to wash before you come', and I find that they more than meet me half-way. They all come in their Sunday clothes and put flowers in their hair. After they've seen me or the nurse they go home and change into working clothes for rubber tapping."

Cicely told George Young, "When Miss Simmonds first came to work out here twelve years ago the infant mortality was three times as high as it is today. The change is largely due to her. That's a remarkable achievement, and she hasn't had much assistance from the doctors. I think she has a persistence and a real flair for her work which is quite unusual. What she does is almost unbelievably good, and it is done at very little expense. I think that her work would provide a model for the establishment of this type of work in many other countries. It's badly needed, and will be for many years to come."

Miss Simmonds had come to Singapore only because she felt like a change, and when she arrived the doctors simply said, "There is the rural area. Do maternal and child health work." She began by going round her area in a lorry with a travelling dispensary. She saw the lie of the land and what the villages were like. There was a certain amount of jungle on Singapore Island and a great deal of rubber plantation, and there were some very remote villages, or *kampongs* as they were called. Some of the villages were Chinese and some were mostly Malay. There were also many Indian workers called "coolie" workers. Miss Simmonds gradually build up a department working in these remote areas. Some of her nurses came from the Mission

Hospital in Singapore, St Andrew's, where there was a Nurses' Training School. Some of them were throwouts from the general hospital. Gradually Miss Simmonds managed to establish centres in five or six of the bigger villages and sub-centres in the smaller ones. The smallest centres of all had just one midwife. Miss Simmonds managed to combine the maternal and child health work in a spectacularly efficient way. At one time more than nine out of ten of all the deliveries were done by her midwives, and most of these women were coming regularly to her antenatal clinics and would then bring the babies for regular supervision to her health centres. She never discharged them at one year old as was the custom in many places. She continued to supervise them, and she would tell the mothers that if there was anything wrong they were never to hesitate to bring the children to see her. She gave minor treatment for diseases as she saw them, and she learnt quickly to recognise beri-beri and more serious cases that should be referred to the doctors at the dispensaries or straight to Cicely at the hospital. After that Cicely often visited her health centres and was impressed with the quality of the relationship that Miss Simmonds had built up with the mothers. "Mother, if you don't do what I tell you for this child, you know what will happen. I won't let you come to the clinic any longer." This was the biggest punishment that she could suggest. She even persuaded the mothers to eat the unpolished rice that would save them from beri-beri. Somehow she managed to persuade them to discover it for themselves. They knew that they were feeling bad and getting swellings and being tired and incompetent. But she led them to realise that they felt better if they ate the unpolished rice.

"But in Singapore, as in Africa," Cicely told George Young, "I feel that insufficient attention is being paid to child health. Our wards are always overcrowded. I often have to send children home long before I am satisfied. Without proper out-patients we have no means of knowing what happens to them afterwards. And since the Municipal Welfare Centres don't supervise children over the age of one year, many of them are not receiving sufficient attention. In the Medical School the students come to my wards for two months in a total of five years' training. Considering that nearly half of the population of Singapore is under the age of fourteen, this just isn't good enough. The number of deaths among children is appalling. What's more, there are no antenatal clinics in the maternity hospitals and there is no follow-up after delivery. The biggest medical need is more attention and care for women and children."

During the late afternoon, as they approached Fraser's Hill, there was a heavy tropical rain-storm. They had to stop the car because of blinding rain on the windscreen. The jungle became darker than ever, and water poured down the tree trunks. Steam rose through the vines and undergrowth that twined round giant trees. Afterwards the silence was broken by water dripping slowly from the leaves and by the occasional call of a bird or the chatter of monkeys.

"My God, you don't believe that, do you?"

The speaker was Jack Scharff, Chief Medical Officer for the rural areas of Singapore and Professor of Public Health in the University. Cicely had become friendly with him through Miss Simmonds.

He happened to be in her office when she received a visitor, an Indian who worked for the American Express and had a Japanese wife. Through Cicely they were arranging to adopt a child which was to be handed over after they had been on a duty visit to Bangkok. His return had been delayed, and he came in to explain that this was because the trains were all occupied by "Japanese farmers" going to South Thailand.

"You mean he's not trustworthy?" Cicely answered absent-mindedly, for she was still thinking about the child. She had found an orphaned baby, half-Indian and half-Japanese, that she thought would suit them. She was suddenly worried that Scharff thought the man was an unsuitable parent.

"That's not what I meant."

There was a silence. Feelings of tension and dread came over

Cicely. She was increasingly familiar with these feelings whenever she stopped thinking about her babies and allowed herself to dwell on wider issues.

"Why on earth should the Japanese send farmers to South Thailand?"

"Anything more bogus I can't imagine. Yet no one is doing anything about it," Scharff continued. "It's plain for all to see that the Japanese are building up troops to invade Malaya overland. Yet everyone, including the authorities, prefers to accept cock and bull stories about 'farmers'."

"And what about the Japanese fishermen?" Cicely knew there were hundreds of these.

"You may well ask. I'm certain that many are spies and agents."

"I've had an ominous feeling about the Japanese ever since I came to the East. It's the sort of thing I have to switch off when it rises in my mind."

"Do you get Japanese children in your hospital?"

"Sometimes. I find them charming beyond words. I'm always struck by the amount of discipline to which they're exposed. Practically as soon as the child can hold his head up he's taught to bow. If you speak to a mother with a baby in her arms she keeps pushing its head down to make it bow."

"What's the reaction of the Chinese nurses?"

"My Chinese amahs are fond of Japanese babies and they call them 'Nippon'. Although the Chinese have a deep, fierce hatred of the Japanese, they don't seem to transfer to the children any of the antagonism that they feel towards their race."

"Everybody tries not to think about it," said Scharff, sadly. "Even the Chinese. Would you care to come with me to see the Japanese warship?"

"The one in Singapore harbour?"

"That's right. They have invited a whole lot of people, including me. My wife's away and you can come in her place. I guarantee that you'll see a demonstration of the iron hand in a velvet glove."

As they went on board a Japanese officer bowed low and handed them a typewritten sheet. It explained in pedantic and idiosyncratic English that the ferocious names of the Japanese warships meant that they were aggressive and deadly. It also informed its readers that the Japanese people were gentle and sweet as the wind. The British guests saw the ship at work and were taken on deck for demonstrations of ju-jitsu, single stick and Japanese wrestling.

"I think these wrestlers are the most revolting human beings I have ever seen," whispered Cicely to Jack Scharff.

"It's the combined demonstration of aggressiveness and suavity that I find terrifying," he said.

As they left he nudged her. "See that Japanese photographer. He's not here just because it happens to be a Japanese ship. The British use him for all their official photographs on both social and official occasions. So he goes round with our blessing, taking photographs of our ships and military installations and so on. What's the betting that when the Japanese finally invade us we shall find that we've given him all the information they need?"

Increasingly Cicely was feeling that the political situation was becoming so difficult that anything might happen. She longed to get away somewhere where she could work without constant political anxiety.

About the time of the Munich crisis she was invited to stay in Hong Kong with Sir Geoffrey and Lady Northcote. Sir Geoffrey had been Colonial Secretary in Ghana and was now Governor of Hong Kong. She decided to go for a month, which was her local leave saved up for two years. She stayed nearly six weeks because she fell sick and had to go to hospital. When she was better she watched the refugees coming over the border, fleeing from the Japanese invasion of South China. More than 50,000 people were sleeping in the streets. When the situation became more tense the Governor moved his family and guests from Mountain Lodge at the top of the peak to Government House in Hong Kong itself. Here Cicely had an interesting time seeing the different provisions that were being made for the refugees and watching the situation between Japan and China and the Hong Kong community develop. As each week passed she felt things getting blacker.

"There's going to be war," said Jack Scharff, when she arrived back in Singapore. "If you take my advice you'll get out before it's too late."

But she was busy digging herself in. She had been offered a flat in the General Hospital, which was more convenient for her work. She felt that her wards needed constant attention at night, which she could not give when she lived two miles away.

The General Hospital had only been built about twelve years previously. It was a good serviceable building. In one block there were two floors, each with two or three flats for medical officers. They were comfortable, with good sitting rooms and balconies and two or three large bedrooms, each with its own bathroom. But when she went to inspect the servants' quarters she found that, though there were excellent rooms for the men-servants and their families, there were no bathrooms for them.

She went to see the Hospital Secretary and complained. He was a quiet little man, perhaps browbeaten, certainly rigid. He told her that there was a bathroom for the servants on the roof and a lavatory on the ground floor.

"But you don't expect the servants to live like that, do you?"

"No doctor has complained before, Dr Williams." He wasn't very interested.

"I don't wonder that the Europeans get worms. If a baby's pants have to be washed, do you suppose that the mother is going up to the roof or down to the basement? No. She'll wash them in the kitchen sink, of course, just where the cook is washing his lettuce."

She refused to move in. The Hospital Secretary didn't seem to care. She took a furnished flat near by and thought that nothing would happen. But eventually all the servants' quarters were altered and supplied with bathrooms. Cicely, with her Malay boy Ali, his wife Mina, and their small son

Fazil, flourished in their new accommodation, and Cicely was relieved to be so near her patients.

In the summer of 1939 there were rumblings of war in Europe. Cicely was nearly exhausted after four years in the children's wards in Singapore. She was beginning to think that it was time to move on again. Her position in the Colonial Service was unsatisfactory. Although she was a qualified specialist with full specialist responsibility, she was not paid or established as such. She resented this, and knew that had she been a man, and if the subject of child health had had any status she would have been in a settled position with twice the salary. She also felt uncertain about the future, feeling that the world might erupt.

She was due for leave to visit her friends in England and her family in Jamaica for perhaps the last time for many years. She booked her passage, handed over her flat and made arrangements for her work to be covered. With the lightheartedness that comes from shedding responsibilities, she went to the Medical Headquarters to say "Goodbye".

The Chief Medical Officer shook her by the hand warmly and said, "You're not going. All leave is cancelled."

Tired and disappointed, she returned to work, living in temporary accommodation until her flat was free. In September war was declared, and a few days later she developed pneumonia. Her health and spirits were low. She would clearly be unfit to work for many weeks. She was told to take leave, but not to go to England.

With an effort she climbed out of her despair and decided to go to Java to study the child health services. Whatever personal and national disaster might come, there were always the children, sick, underfed and visibly in need of her services. The more she could travel and see what was going on in different countries, the more valuable she would be wherever she worked.

She returned to Singapore restored in health, and decided to resign from the Colonial Service and go and work in India. Conditions for women doctors were much better there, and she was offered a post as paediatrician to the Dufferin Hospital in Calcutta. She was very much looking forward to her new life. But before leaving Malaya finally she agreed to go north for a few weeks, to help her friend Jack Scharff.

"Your job," said the Sultan of Trengganu to Cicely, "is to improve the health of mothers and babies."

They were drinking tea together in the cool, dark palace. The Sultan was clever and vigorous, much influenced by Jack Scharff, whom he liked. Through Scharff's influence the Sultan invited Cicely first to do a survey of child health and later to take over for six months from Dr Leslie Shield, the Chief Medical Officer of Trengganu, during his six months' leave. She managed to get leave from the Medical School and University in Singapore and travelled on the railway that runs up the centre of the Malay peninsula towards Kelantan. The railway station was a hundred miles from the capital, Kuala Trengganu, and here she was met by her friend George de Moubray, who was the British Resident, and his wife Katherine, who invited her to stay. Both were good Malay scholars with great experience in Malaya, devoted to the people and much admired by them.

Trengganu is in the north-west of Malaya, just south of Kelantan, which reaches the border of Thailand. Cicely instantly loved the beautiful country. The coast was lined with rocks and palms, and by miles of paddy fields and bright sandy beaches, often separated by rocks covered with trees and foliage. Inland a mountain range ran southwards, and mountains and jungle sloped down towards the China Sea. Much of the land was uninhabited. The people mostly lived along the coast and worked as fishermen. There was little cattle farming, but they grew rice and coconuts. They made beautiful boats, curved, pointed at both ends, made without nails, and called "the one day moon". The wood was bent by being steamed over a fire, and holes were drilled for wooden pegs. They also wove beautiful silk sarongs and cotton, and made many of their own patterns. And they produced a sort of metal work from which they made domestic articles, including the dainty little sets used for chewing betel. There were small containers for nuts, lime, spices and betel leaf.

"And what's more," said the Sultan, in his colloquial English, "I expect you to do it at no cost. Of course you realise we have no money."

"Of course," smiled Cicely, knowing that at least Dr Scharff had already engaged a Chinese health visitor, Miss Kee, who had had excellent experience in Penang.

"There is a great deal to do."

"Of course," smiled Cicely again, suspecting how much of an understatement this was.

She was the only European doctor in the state. She had under her three other doctors, two Chinese and an Indian. There were no trained nurses but several midwives. There was a hospital of about 160 beds in Kuala Trengganu, and four other hospitals in some of the bigger villages. Dressers or medical assistants were stationed in other places.

The state of Trengganu was even more backward than other Malayan states. It was probably the first part of the mainland to be converted to the Moslem faith in the thirteenth century. With the help of the three other doctors she would be in charge of as many as 300,000 people, most of them Moslem Malays. There were few Chinese except in the bigger towns, and only a few Indians. In the south were a few large estates. Some iron mines were actually owned by Japanese, and most of the employees on these mines were Chinese. There were also one or two tin mines which employed Chinese labourers.

On her second afternoon Cicely took over the bungalow belonging to the medical officer, who was on leave. It was comfortable and close to the hospital, with telephone and electric light. None of the other houses had electricity, but the M.O.'s bungalow enjoyed the hospital's electricity supply.

That evening she was lying on the sofa reading when she noticed bullet holes scattered across the wooden roof. She asked the houseboy how they had got there, and was told that one of the previous medical officers used to lie on the sofa in the sitting room and practise shooting with his revolver, aiming at the lizards in the roof. She noticed that there were also bullet holes in the door of the bathroom. The boy told her that these had been produced on one particular occasion. Every year there was a formal dinner party for all the Europeans, about twelve in the whole state. But they tended to regard this ritual party with some foreboding because it lasted a long time and meant sitting on the floor and eating with the fingers, and, as it was a Moslem state, there was no alcohol. The wife of one of the Government servants had tried to keep the men in order, so that they would arrive at the dinner party clean and tidy. She and her husband, a police officer, had gone to the M.O.'s bungalow to take him to dinner. They discovered him sitting in the little green tin bath. On the back of the bathroom door he had pinned a picture of a pink elephant. He had his gun on his knees and was taking pot shots at the picture of the pink elephant.

Cicely was never bored in Trengganu. She soon became known as "Tuan Mem Doktah Besar", which means "Lord High Female Doctor". She and Miss Kee, the Chinese health nurse, started work with a vigour and vision such as had not been seen before in the state.

The Malays were a big problem. They were difficult to reach and resistant to European medicine. Cicely and her staff arranged for a small hut to be built not far from the hospital, because they knew that the women and children would be unwilling to come to the hospital itself at first. To get themselves known she and Miss Kee went visiting in the town, asking the mothers to bring their babies. They were also able to use a Malay men's club, where they held sessions on Sundays.

Miss Kee did much visiting in the town. She went to all the houses where there were newborn babies and encouraged the mothers to bring their children to the clinic. They started another centre at the dispensary inside the town which was a little way from the hospital. Cicely was delighted to see how rapidly the people began to respond, both Chinese and Malays. Miss Kee persuaded all the men who worked in the hospital, from the senior clerk down to the most junior man in the kitchen, to bring their wives and children to her clinics. This was a useful form of attack because they were intelligent, educated and responsive. It soon became the done thing to take your children to Miss Kee every week, and the men learnt to appreciate the value of her supervision. There was soon a marked difference between the children who had been brought up, as they used to say, "before Miss Kee", and the ones who were "with Miss Kee".

"I would never have thought it possible to control bed bugs," said Ho Ching, the senior hospital clerk, admiringly. Cicely, who was in charge of the hospital, had made massive war on these ubiquitous creatures.

"I don't think we'll ever eliminate them," she said. "But at least we've shown that we can reduce their numbers considerably. It's not difficult if you're determined. Actually I find the food question more difficult." One of her duties was to supervise the hospital food. "It's so difficult to find food that is acceptable to all three races."

"This has always been a problem to us," said Ho Ching. He was an elderly and still handsome Chinese, grizzled, wise and friendly. Cicely liked him.

"Another thing that worries me," she went on, "is that we have so many Chinese patients in the hospital. Although the Chinese community is small here in Kuala Trengganu it provides most of our patients."

"The Chinese take better to European medicine. But there are plenty of Indian patients too."

"Yes, but few Malays, although nearly all the people in the town and round about are Malay. It's very worrying."

Ho Ching looked at her with interest and approval but shrugged his shoulders. "Most Malays are simple people and shy about participating in Western medicine."

"That's why their mortality rate is so dreadful."

She thought about the problem deeply. Miss Kee was already doing excellent work. Dr Scharff, during his stay, had also done much to make life more healthy for the Malays, and for this he had three main lines of attack. One was improving the Public Health organisation in the town itself and in some of the villages round, improving the water supply, protecting rivers and springs, and controlling malaria by subsoil drainage, by oiling and spraying mosquito breeding places and by collecting rubbish. He also organised the making of compost and encouraged people to grow more vegetables to vary the agriculture. His third approach was to try to persuade the people to eat under-milled rice. At that time Malaya grew only one-third of the total rice it consumed. Much rice was grown in Trengganu, but most of what was eaten was cheap polished rice from Siam. This caused many cases of beri-beri.

Soon after Dr Scharff arrived he had started a Government mill. He persuaded people to bring their rice, and showed them how to do the milling in the right way to produce rice which still had a large quantity of vitamin B_1. Cicely knew that authorities were wrong who said it was impossible to make people change from eating white rice to eating under-milled rice. In a short time so many people brought their rice to the Government mill that it could no longer cope with the demand. It was clear that acceptable education spread rapidly.

Determined to improve the health of the Malays still further, Cicely began to make excursions with Miss Kee out of the town to the outlying villages to assess the health of the people and the amount of malaria, yaws and other indigenous diseases. All along the coast rivers ran down from the mountains into the sea, and none of the rivers had any real bridges. Travelling north and south, which was practically the only direction of the motor roads, meant crossing these rivers. Cicely suffered anxiety about this. She found it terrifying to drive her car backwards down two boards on to the ferry boat, and was convinced that one day she would end up in the water.

Sometimes she went out in a boat because her domain included islands along the coast. When the work was finished they usually bathed off the boat in the glorious clear tropical sea with the most amazing underwater shells and seaweeds and anemones.

Motor roads were few, and to reach some of the villages they had to walk for miles. Some of the people in these villages had never seen a white woman. As soon as Cicely appeared everyone would go into their houses and the village became like a city of the dead. But Cicely felt that their reluctance to appear was due to a conventional shyness rather than to fear. She and Miss Kee would go to the *wakaf* in the middle of the village. *Wakafs* were semi-religious shelters built by Malays, often at cross-roads, where you could sit and rest on your journey. People went there to pray or gossip, and it made a useful place of meeting or shelter. The two women would sit there and eat coconuts or sugar cane. Gradually children would come and peer, and slowly inquisitiveness overcame shyness. Usually two or three children started to peep. Then they would come close enough to smile, and would want to come and touch Cicely. Her red hair and white skin intrigued them, and they wanted to feel if it was real. Other children would follow, and then the grownups. Once the barrier was broken she could feel their tummies to see if they had enlarged spleens or livers from malaria. Sometimes she could examine as many as 200 children in a single village, looking for large spleens, for anaemia, for yaws and for all the obvious manifestations of the local diseases. After the children had shown the way the adults followed. First the men came one by one, often straight from the fields or from fishing. When the women saw the men coming they too would follow, and before long they invited the strangers to their houses and showed them where the rice was stored, how the cooking was done and the other things they wanted to know. Then, of course, they would show them the grandmother who was sick and couldn't get up, and the child who had severe fever and other problems. While wandering in the villages Cicely learnt much about the way of life.

She was happy in Trengganu, partly because adventures sometimes developed in the simplest way, such as over the question of drinking milk.

She had long been concerned about milk. The damage caused by tinned milk to the children of Singapore had affected her deeply, and wherever she went she looked out for supplies of fresh animal milk. In Trengganu milk was scarce. A few cows wandered in the compounds and between the paddy fields, poor little things with little milk. But everwhere were buffaloes, huge, solid, pulling primitive ploughs.

One day Cicely went to an agricultural show with an able young health inspector from Singapore. They saw prizes given for handsome buffaloes, for ploughing and for hauling timber.

"Do the people ever drink buffalo milk?" she asked suddenly. The agricultural officer, who had lived there for many years, shook his head.

"I'm sure they don't. Why do you ask?"

"It suddenly occurred to me. Buffalo milk is concentrated. It has a high fat content and is extremely nourishing. It's unsuitable for small babies, but it's splendid for a child of toddler age or for anyone else."

"I'm sure they only use buffaloes for ploughing and heavy work."

But she wasn't convinced. She had seen *ghee* on sale, and knew that this was clarified butter. She could not think how they got it except from the buffaloes. The health inspector promised to make enquiries.

A few days later he came back and said, "No, they don't."

"Well, we'll go on finding out," said Cicely with determination.

A few days later he came and said, "You were right. They do drink buffaloes' milk but they're ashamed of it. They say that nice people in the towns drink milk from a tin, not milk from the behind of a buffalo."

"I'd like to make certain."

"All right. We'll go out one morning."

They rose about four o'clock one morning and went to some of the *kampongs*. At first no one seemed to be milking buffaloes. Eventually they found an old man in a buffalo pen which protected the animals from tigers at night. He was milking a buffalo, and since there was no question of concealing it he was communicative. He showed them how they milked the buffaloes into bamboo joints, and he said that this buffalo cow gave one joint full, that one two or three joints full, and so on.

"What do you do with the milk?" asked Cicely.

"I drink it," he said. "It makes me strong." And he bulged his biceps.

"Do you ever give it to the women or children?"

"Certainly not. What I don't drink we sell. The women curdle it and sell it in the market."

"Is milking a woman's work? Do women ever milk the buffaloes?"

"No," he said. "That would be impossible."

Cicely and her friend moved on to the farm next door and found a woman milking buffaloes.

"This," said Cicely, triumphantly, "is what you call research."

Later they went to the market and found that what the old man had said was true. But the buffalo *sapi* or yoghurt was always kept under the counter because of shyness about admitting that one drank buffaloes' milk.

She discovered that people who had buffaloes always milked them and drank the milk either fresh or as curds. She was able to order bamboos full of buffalo milk for her hospital. She wanted to persuade the patients to drink it and to adopt it as part of their diet. She walked up and down her wards with a bamboo of curds in one hand and a teaspoon in the other, eating in front of the patients and saying that anybody who liked could have some. The demand turned out to be quite brisk, and in a remarkably short time it seemed possible to convince people that it was not shameful to drink buffaloes' milk. She arranged for samples of it to be shown in the clinics, and the mothers were taught how to mix it with rice porridge for the toddler children who, as in all tropical countries, were the worst fed of all.

They started to train nurses and midwives, and Cicely was anxious that during their training these students should go out into the villages. She wanted them to be independent and mobile. There was also a dentist and she wanted him not merely to sit in the hospital and attend to people's teeth, but to go out into the schools and give lectures on the care of teeth and inspect the school children and identify those who needed treatment. But it was difficult to move about. Cars were expensive, and few people could afford them. It occurred to Cicely that on many of the village pathways it would be possible to bicycle between the paddy fields. She suggested to the authorities that a few bicycles would greatly improve the work, but she was told that it would be improper for senior officers to ride bicycles.

So she ordered a bicycle for herself from Singapore. She had not ridden one since she was at Oxford twenty years previously, but she was determined to show that senior officers could ride bicycles. She would bicycle from the hospital into the town and inspect the collection of rubbish and then, as conspicuously as possible, would visit the more important shopping areas and the schools. It caused quite a sensation among the people, but it was clear that she would have to prove her point more impressively if the authorities were to be induced to provide bicycles for the nurses and midwives. She felt that if she could show direct benefit the battle might be won.

Eventually she thought of the solution. The authorities were keen on cleanliness and tidiness, and waged constant war on litter and those who caused it. There was one particular offender. He sold a popular form of beverage from a handcart on which he carried much sugar cane. He pushed the handcart along grinding the sugar cane, and the juice was collected in tumblers and sold for a few cents a tumblerful. Each time he ground a piece of sugar cane, he flung the trash into the street. Cicely pursued him through the streets on her bicycle and made him reverse his journey, picking up every bit of cane trash that he had dropped. She had won her point and the bicycles were ordered.

She spent some time helping to teach the nurses and midwives to ride the bicycles, and managed to arrange for an increase in pay as soon as they had learnt the art. At first it was considered impossible for women to ride bicycles, but within a few weeks there was an enthusiastic group of nurses who were proud of their bicycles and of their agility. Now they could move about quickly and independently among the *kampongs*.

She also started regular lectures for the staff, and a rotation system by which some of the dressers went into the *kampongs* to work and then came back to Kuala Trengganu for certain periods. There was great enthusiasm for the lectures, and Cicely was asked to have them typed and circulated. In this way, even those who were away in the *kampongs* could keep in touch with the courses.

And so the days passed, busy, purposeful, often amusing and always interesting. Like everyone else Cicely knew that the war was approaching and that one day they might be invaded by the Japanese. Everyone carried on as usual and tried not to think about it. The Allies had no troops stationed in Trengganu, but there were a few further north in Kelantan, and sometimes the officers came over for discussions with the British residents. The Malays much admired the army vehicles which occasionally drove into the town.

"If war comes," said Cicely cheerfully to Miss Kee, "I'm certain that the Malays will use camouflage as one of the patterns in their home-woven sarongs. They are so skilful at adapting anything topical into their weaving."

Later it seemed to her curious that they had all been so detached.

She was supposed to be in Trengganu until the end of August, 1941, when Dr Leslie Shield was coming back from his vacation in New Zealand. She had now heard that she had been confirmed in the coveted post as paediatrician to the Dufferin Hospital in Calcutta, and she had permission to resign from the Colonial Service. But shortly before Dr Shield's return she received an urgent request from the Sultan in Council to stay on in Trengganu. Everyone was so pleased with her work that they were willing to find salaries for both her and Dr Shield. They wanted her to stay for another three years to develop the work in maternal and child health that she had started. Cicely explained that she had already accepted the post in Calcutta and therefore could not stay so long. But she agreed to stay for three months.

Those three months led to her undoing.

CHAPTER VII

On 8 December, 1941, Cicely came down to breakfast with even more than usual on her mind. Her work in Trengganu was shaping its own rewards. People in positions of authority were beginning to take her seriously. This morning she was going to see George de Moubray, the British Advisor, who was keen to see plans of how to extend her work. She could already feel into the future to a time of safe childhood, with healthy, educated mothers and thousands of flourishing babies growing up all over the state, well fed and protected from crippling diseases of ignorance and prejudice.

She switched on the radio and reached for the toast, but her hand stopped on its way. A voice, sombre and controlled but with unconcealed emotion, hit her like a physical blow.

"The Japanese have landed at Kota Bahru and fighting is going on."

Like everyone else, she had been expecting it for at least two years. Yet it seemed that the heavens had fallen.

She left her breakfast untouched and hurried to the hospital. It seemed to be more silent than usual. Staff and walking patients moved about uneasily, almost furtively, hurrying without purpose and clustering near the few radio sets. There were no special orders except to carry on with normal work.

"How far is Kota Bahru?"

"About 100 miles north of here."

"Not far for an army."

"They'll be here any day."

News came over the air from Singapore and Penang but it was difficult to make sense of it.

"What's happening? Why don't they tell us?"

"Probably no one knows. After a landing of this sort the fighting is always confused."

"If the invasion succeeds, what will become of us?"

"God knows. Anything. But one thing is certain. There's not a hope of holding Trengganu."

"Oh God," screamed someone. "They're here. The Japanese are marching down the street."

Anguished, they rushed to the windows. Half a dozen police were marching a column of men down the street. They were Japanese. There was a moment's silence, then someone said, "They're only the local residents going off to be interned."

Immense relief. One or two people tittered. They knew that there were about sixty Japanese left in the state of Trengganu, most of them in the tin mines. The rest had been ordered back to Japan some months before.

"Quiet, please. There's some more news."

The contained voice of the announcer from Singapore was clearly audible. "Since our last bulletin, half-an-hour ago . . ." The voice was drowned in a burst of melody.

"What on earth is that music?"

"*Keep the Home Fires Burning!*"

"What does it mean? Why do they play it?"

"God knows. A signal, perhaps."

Years later they learnt that it had been a signal from the Japanese in Saigon.

"It's eerie."

"One's so helpless."

"Not as helpless as the patients. At least we can use our legs if need be."

"Legs! Where will our legs carry us?"

"We must carry on with our work as best we can."

"Discharge all patients who can possibly leave."

"We can't move Yen Pi. She's lost too much blood. If she is sent away she will die and probably her baby too."

"There's *Keep the Home Fires Burning* again. It gives me the creeps."

The next few days were confused, and it was difficult to keep track of what was happening. On the third day Penang fell. The British Advisor came to the hospital and announced that

Trengganu would not be defended. No one was surprised. Everyone was outwardly calm.

"What will happen to the Europeans?" At last someone voiced the unspoken question.

They all knew that the Europeans would be ordered to leave, because if they stayed the local people might have a worse time than if the Japanese took over without disrupting the territory.

"We'll let you know as soon as we know ourselves."

Then followed a whole day of discussions, because the British Advisor was ordered to try to persuade the Sultan to retire from the state before the Japanese arrived, and not to treat with the enemy. The Sultan arrived at the Residency bringing his household in fifteen cars. It was obvious that such an entourage could not withdraw very far.

While the rumours scuttled backwards and forwards Cicely worked on, treating her patients. The idea of leaving them became increasingly impossible. She had overwhelming feelings that her duty was to remain at work as long as she possibly could. Katherine de Moubray had similar feelings, and also stayed.

One afternoon at lunchtime a messenger burst into the doctors' room in the hospital, and announced, "The Japanese are advancing from Besut in the north and have also landed at Kuantan in the south."

There was silence and shock. Then someone said nervously, "Can we get to the railway?"

"Not a chance. That road goes north and must be cut off by now, like the road to Kuantan."

"Could we go down the coast?"

"There's no road."

"It seems extraordinary," someone burst out angrily. "They haven't built even a track down the coast in this God-forsaken country."

"The explanation is simple," said a calmer voice. "In Malaya roads were built to serve the railway rather than to compete with it or to duplicate it."

"What a time to lecture!" said someone else. "Isn't there anything else we can do?"

"The only alternative is to trek over the mountains and go down the centre of the peninsula until we can join the railway."

"Could we do that?"

"God knows. The mountains are formidable."

"We should also have to get through the jungle, which is even worse than the mountains."

"What about going by river?"

"Difficult. The river beds are full of snags and fallen timber. And you can't go across the peninsula by river because the chief streams run longitudinally."

"What about further up?"

"That would be difficult too. There are rapids all over the place."

The information about the double Japanese advance turned out to be false, but not before they had all acted upon it.

By three o'clock that afternoon the Sultan had decided to leave with the British Advisor and Katherine de Moubray, and to take his entire suite up the Trengganu river to Kuala Berang and from there to cross the mountains into Pahang. De Moubray did not approve of this route, so he told the rest of the Europeans to get out by the Dungun river. He divided them into two parties. In one, two men were to go south with some Malay policemen and a few other people to pick up the women who had already started, and also the other Europeans in Dungun. They were to take them up the Dungun river to join the rest of the party, who were to go by road to Jerangau, which was farther up the river. The people from Dungun were to organise boats to take everyone up the river and into the mountains. They would cross over by the divide and climb down the other side of the mountain range to a place called Kuala Lipis, where they would take a train.

It was an ambitious scheme, and even Cicely, usually so fearless, found the thought of the journey frightening. The path through the jungle had once been travelled by two Europeans in the dry season. It was now wet and the rivers were high.

There was no path and no road. People merely knew the general direction. You went up the mountain and down the other side. As long as you were going up you were going in the right direction. No woman had ever made this journey before.

"How can I leave my patients?" she asked, in miserable indecision. "They need me, some of them even for their lives. Yet anyone who conceals me may get into terrible trouble." The thought of what the Japanese might do to her Malay or Chinese friends made the situation unbearable.

"Don't go, Miss Doctor," said Ho Ching, the senior clerk of the hospital, a Chinese whom Cicely greatly admired. "We need you here," he said. "We can protect you through the immediate crisis without much danger either to you or to ourselves. Some of us are sending our wives to *kampongs* in the jungle. You can go with them and stay hidden there. We will fetch you when the trouble is over."

"But what if you are found concealing me?" she asked, finding it hard to control her voice.

He smiled with confidence. "We won't be caught," he said quietly.

She believed him, and so her only reason for leaving was gone. She went to find Leslie Shield, the Chief Medical Officer, to tell him that she had decided to stay. She expected to find him packing to leave with the rest of the Europeans, but he was sitting behind his desk. He listened to what she had to say and answered in a quiet imperative.

"I'm sorry, Cicely. I'm ordering you to leave and I myself am going to stay," he said.

"This is absurd," cried Cicely. "You are a strong young man. You can go into the Army. If I stay here I am no loss to anybody and I can carry on and look after the patients."

"I'm not arguing," he said, quietly. "I'm giving you orders. Time is short."

She had to give in. There seemed no alternative. As she left his office she could hear the sound of rioting in the streets, and she suddenly wondered why no attempt had been made to hand over to Malays the control of the police, prisons and other instruments of public order. Astonishingly, the police and volunteers had been disbanded and prisoners released. As a result there was stampeding, looting and general disorder throughout the town.

In contemplating the hazardous journey across the peninsula Cicely realised she had other responsibilities too. One was a Malay nurse from Singapore who had no relatives in Trengganu. She had never done any walking, and it was unlikely that she could manage a long trek of this sort. Also, if they were overtaken by Japanese it would be more dangerous for her to be caught with the crowd of Europeans. Cicely decided that on the whole it would be better to risk allowing her to stay in the *kampongs* with the other nurses than to attempt to take her through the jungle. Finally she arranged for her to stay in Kuala Trengganu with a Malay family who said that they would protect her. By a curious coincidence Cicely met the nurse in Borneo after the war and so discovered that she had survived.

Another problem was a Chinese amah called Ah Yong, whose home was in Ipoh on the other side of the peninsula. She asked to go with the European party because she had no Chinese friends in Trengganu.

Everyone seemed to be crying, and it was difficult not to do the same. The realisation that the Europeans were really fleeing seemed suddenly to bring the situation home to the hospital staff, who had hitherto kept fear at bay by preoccupation with their patients' needs in the emergency.

"What will become of us if you go?" wailed a Chinese ward sister. Her tense white face haunted Cicely for months afterwards. Everyone knew that the Japanese would treat the Chinese more harshly than they would treat the Malays.

"I must take medical supplies," answered Cicely, struggling back to a practical level. "See, I have brought a haversack. I shall be the only doctor in the party."

But she was still unconvinced that she would really go, and almost automatically she wandered to Leslie Shield's office for another attempt to persuade him to change places with her.

"As a man," she pleaded, "you would be of more use in the defence of Malaya than I would be. And as a woman I shall probably receive better treatment from the Japanese if I stay behind to work in the hospital."

"No, Cicely, I'm sorry. It's out of the question. Now hurry." He turned away, tired and tense. "Go and collect your belongings. Time is short. Whatever have you got in that rucksack?"

"Medical supplies. I've just collected them in the hospital."

"You'll never be able to carry all that. You'll have your own things too."

"I must take drugs and dressings. They are more important than my personal belongings. Maybe we'll find porters."

"Do you never think of yourself, Cicely?"

"Coming from you in the present situation, Leslie, that's a strange question." Her own voice sounded distant and unfamiliar to her.

"Perhaps we'll meet again one day. Goodbye, Cicely."

Outside the door she met Saleh, Shield's boy, and his remark hurt her more than anything she had encountered during those confused and frightening days.

"Of course, my *master* is not going to run away."

The feeling roused in Cicely was one of deep and burning shame.

There was a last meeting at the British Resident's house, and the Director of Education, a Malay, was there. He was friendly, and the only person who managed to cheer Cicely up.

"Don't worry," he said. "It can't last long. In a couple of weeks you'll be back. Don't worry about us, we'll carry on meanwhile."

"You must leave your car," she was told. "Please lock it and throw away the key."

Sadly she stroked her car on its familiar red roof. She was fond of it. Then she threw the key far into the jungle in a final act of hope and despair.

She began the long journey as the passenger in a car driven by a genial administrative officer called Cobden Ramsey, who had been second in command to the British Advisor. He started by driving back towards the town to pick up a man called Jerram and to buy food for the journey. To their relief, the grocer's shop was still open. They bought some rice and a dozen tins of different foods and stowed it all in the car. They could not find Jerram, and it was too dangerous to wait for him. So after a last search they turned the car round and headed out of the town.

It was about forty-five miles to Jerangau. The first part was on a good road up towards Kuala Berang. Everywhere were signs of people racing away from the town and cars overturned. The last thirty miles were along a practically unused road through a forest reserve. Twice the car got stuck in the mud and they had to push it out. It was getting late, and it was an area with many tigers.

They reached Jerangau at sunset. A Chinese shop on the river provided coffee in a dark little room with an earth floor and dogs, chickens and children. The villagers were friendly and anxious to help.

Two motorboats arrived from Dungun. Cicely and Cobden Ramsey learnt that the men had got through all right and picked up the women, and also an Australian called Macvilly. This party had come up by a difficult overland route, walking most of the night. They were now waiting upstream.

After initial greetings Cicely was conscious of rising tension between the men. Personalities clashed in an undercurrent of fear. Arguments grew into recriminations. Everyone was nervous, and even the air seemed jittery. She decided to camp in one of the boats. Later two of the men, Reece and Paterson, joined her, and said that the atmosphere in the men's dormitory was uncongenial.

Next morning at dawn they started off in the motorboats, and by midday had reached the *kampong* where they had arranged to pick up the other members of the party.

"Where on earth can they be?" There was no sign of Europeans, only silent Malays and frightened children running in the dust.

"We'll wait awhile," said Cobden Ramsey, and they stretched themselves out on the river bank. Presently white men emerged through the jungle. They had hidden when they heard the motor boats coming because they did not know whether it was their friends or the Japanese.

It was the rainy season and the river was full. But by the afternoon they had reached a place where the larger boat could go no further. After a short stop the women and the luggage were put into the smaller boat, and the men had a long walk through the jungle to the next stop, a *kampong* near a mine. There was a shop and a house, and the occupants cooked rice and curry for the party. They bought eggs and tins of pilchards, and ate a large meal. In the evening they held council and appointed Cobden Ramsey as chairman.

There were several alternative routes which they might take, and not everyone agreed. But after some discussion they decided that they would all move on as quickly as possible, and try to cross the mountains to reach Kuala Lipis and the railway. They split into three parties to avoid unwieldiness and friction. In the first party strong young men would hurry ahead to bring back help for the rest. Since only two Europeans had ever made this journey before, everyone felt that it was dangerous. Some expressed doubts as to whether the women would be able to manage at all. This first party was led by Brant, an efficient District Officer from Dungun, who turned out to be a good organiser. He took with him three other Europeans and two Malays who had been ordered to join the party. Cicely felt that it was extremely decent of them to obey. They had left their wives and families behind them, and they were grim with anxiety.

The second party consisted of women with their husbands and other willing helpers. Macvilly, the Australian, went with this party to give them extra help.

Everyone else went in the third party. It was considered important that Cicely, as the only doctor, should bring up the rear so that any sickness or accidents in the two forward groups could be left behind for her to deal with. This party had to carry extra food, blankets and medical stores. It contained Cobden Ramsey and March, the District Officer from Besut, who had already done a big job in destroying petrol and other stores. There was also the missing Jerram, who had joined the party from another car. He was an Australian Survey Officer, tall, emaciated and subject to gastritis, which was entirely cured on the jungle diet of rice and tinned food, but reappeared as soon as they reached civilisation. Katagisu was a Tamil Surveyor who was trying to get back to his family in Kuala Lumpur. Machado, the Eurasian headmaster of the English school in Kuala Trengganu, was trying to return to his unit in Singapore.

There was also Ah Yong, the amah, a small woman of about fifty, always neat, sweet, hardworking and cheerful. The party was completed by two European men and two Chinese women, who were nothing but a hindrance and a source of friction. Fortunately, with the exception of one of the men, before long they all went their separate ways.

On the Friday morning they divided their assets and re-packed their luggage. They had only about twenty tins between them. The first and second parties took a few and Cicely's party carried the rest, including anything that might be useful for invalid diets. As an expedition they were poorly equipped. They had bought some extra tins of milk and sardines at the shop, but most of these were stolen before they even arrived at the boats. They had also bought some extra rice and shoes. Cicely had been lucky here. Originally she had had nothing suitable for trekking. She had to leave all her clothes and toilet things behind in Kuala Trengganu except for a pair of dark blue slacks, a shirt and a couple of sarongs and comb, toothbrush, towel and blanket. She insisted on carrying with her her report on the work in Trengganu, some notes for a paper on rickets and a mosquito net. She was able to buy a pair of white canvas rubber-soled shoes, and other members of the expedition gave her a pair of golf stockings, a shirt, a large handkerchief and a pair of khaki shorts. She packed her belongings in a small canvas bag and rolled it in the blanket.

The ends were tied with bandages, and she carried the whole roll over her shoulders with the bandages crossed over her chest and tied behind. She found that she could carry about 15 lb. on her shoulders, and in this way kept her bundle out of the water when they were wading up the rivers. For meals she had a bakelite tumbler and a pocket knife. Between the whole party they had five enamel mugs and one spoon, and there were two other pocket knives and a parang. There was one kettle which leaked after two days. After that all the cooking was done in a big priok, a brass cooking pot which the carriers brought for cooking rice and boiling water.

Late that morning they left Jonka Batu in what was certainly the largest armada ever to set out from there. It was difficult to get three large boats with enough skilled boatmen, and the three parties set out at intervals. They made sure that party No. 1 was the strongest and fastest. The boats were nearly flat-bottomed, each manned by three men. To the amusement of the boatmen Cicely insisted on taking an occasional turn at the punting in her Cherwell style. As a result, at the end of the day she was less stiff than the other members of the party. Occasionally, in the shallows, everyone had to get out and push.

There was little sign of habitation, but Cicely thought it was a lovely winding stream in spite of the overhanging branches and shallow patches due to fallen trees. One of the boatmen, a large and cheerful Tamil, had an almost African smile, though his punting was forceful rather than skilful, and in some ways the trip seemed to her more like a river party than a desperate attempt to escape from an unpleasant death.

Progress was slow. They had hoped to reach Kampong Raja that night, but when darkness came they were still several miles down the river. They had no lights and could see neither the bends in the river nor the snags in their path. At last, cramped and weary with sitting, they saw a fire on a sandy stretch and they heard people shouting.

They moored the boats. Beside the fire was a large cauldron of rice, roasted "stink fish" and banana leaves for use as plates.

Cicely found the meal delicious. It was very dark, and afterwards she bathed in the river in a sarong. Then she and the other women slept uncomfortably in one of the boats under a mosquito net, listening to the chatting, snoring and spitting of the boatmen who slept close by. The mosquitoes buzzed round outside and the sand-flies tormented them inside the net. Some distance away the men had found shelter for themselves in a near-by mosque.

Next morning before dawn she climbed over the side of the boat and walked upstream for another bathe. In spite of all that had happened and was still happening she could yet find pleasure in swimming in the early morning. And here there was the added excitement that one might see a tiger. When day came and the mists had risen she could see that the hills had fallen back and that they were in a wide valley with more cultivation than lower down. But the river was too shallow for the fully laden boats, so after breakfast they all walked a couple of miles over a short cut and the boats followed with the luggage to Kampong Raja itself. By the time Cicely arrived with her party the rest had organised the village into producing roast chicken, boiled rice, eggs and bananas. No. 1 party was already departing, and although it started to rain No. 2 party followed in about an hour, taking all the Malay carriers they could find. From here the journey was to be on foot, and as they did not wish to travel all together Cicely's party decided to rest for another day and give the others a good start.

"Why is it so difficult to get carriers?" someone asked. "There are lots of men in the villages, yet none are willing."

The prospect of carrying their own packs across the mountains loomed large and disquieting.

"I think it's partly a question of health," said Cicely. "They probably don't feel up to it. These up-country Malays are small and wiry, but they are also sick and unenterprising. They're full of worms and yaws and malaria."

"What's more," said the Tamil surveyor, "this is their paddy reaping season and they are all extremely busy."

"Another thing I've noticed," said Ah Yong quietly to Cicely after the men had moved away, "is that there are very few children in these parts."

"The people don't seem to have many," said Cicely. "They only produce about three each, and many die. Also, they keep changing their wives and husbands." She had heard previously about the infertility and matrimonial habits of the mountain Malays.

"We may not be able to find carriers," said Cobden Ramsey, returning from the village, "but at least we've found guides. Apparently some men keep wives on the other side of the mountain, and they like to go over occasionally. They say that there is no actual path but they know the general direction. But . . ." and he stretched himself to his full length in the air as though seeking enjoyment, "I suggest that before we set out we all retire to the *wakaf* for a last binge. Let's eat a leisurely meal and enjoy the rustic landscape."

The *wakaf* was rather superior, a small empty Malay hut on stilts about 4 feet off the ground. In the corner was a fireplace, a large box full of ashes on top of which they lit the fire to cook the rice and chickens they had managed to buy. The ventilation was good, provided by the spaces in the walls and floors. The view was of a pleasant valley with open grazing spaces, buffalo wandering in and about the river and the river winding all among the scenery. Little Malay huts were tucked in among the fruit trees and the bushes. The river up here was too small for navigation, just a stream where they could sit on the sandbanks and wander about knee deep in the water.

Later that day the *penghulu* (head man) brought boiled rice and curry so hot that Cicely could only look at it and weep. He sat with Cobden and discussed the situation. It took a good deal of explanation, but the *penghulu* had heard of "Itu Hitler" (that Hitler). Cicely felt surprised that his remote existence should be affected by such things.

In the morning the baggage problem was serious. The shortage of carriers made it obvious that they would have to carry their own packs. Such Malays as they had been able to enlist would carry the food and the haversack of medical stores. In the morning Cobden gave away three of his service rifles to the *penghulu* and his friends to shoot tiger, elephant and wild pig. He kept a 12-bore which was his favourite, and two of the other men kept service rifles. Cicely wondered whether they were preparing for sport or war.

If she were to succeed in crossing the mountain range she would have to carry as little as possible, and, although she had already sorted through her belongings with this in mind, she did it yet once more. She cast out everything possible, including most of her papers, her satin nightgown and, most painful of all, a shagreen and silver mirror and a little West African leather box that she had had for years. This was no time for sentimentality.

By eight o'clock the guides and carriers had arrived and the loads were distributed. Nearly everyone carried their packs in Malay fashion but the amah, Ah Yong, was different. She found a pole which she carried across her shoulders. At one end were all her possessions, in Cicely's old attaché case, which she said would keep them dry. At the other end she carried a kerosene tin containing tins and precious odds and ends.

In this way she travelled up rivers, through jungles and over mountains, often walking where the rest were crawling on all fours. She never flagged and always trotted along with a smile, in black coat and trousers rolled up at the knees. Her hair was always shining and neat and her expression gentle and demure.

The mists were lifting as they started out. They walked sometimes on a rough track along the river bank and sometimes wading through the shallows, through bits of straggling cultivation which looked as though it had been laid out in extreme absentmindedness. Cicely was surprised at the number of buffalo wallows that always seemed to lie in their path. The guide was a rather dapper Malay with neatly cut hair and a smart striped shirt and shorts. He carried a sarong which went round his head, shoulders or waist, according to requirements. The other Malays were typical jungle people with straggly hair, almost black skinned, small and wiry, with rather Neanderthal features and deeply stained teeth. They were capable of great endurance for a short while, but not of sustained effort, and were unable to carry loads of more than about twenty or thirty pounds. Their dress consisted of a sort of vest and a short sarong with another slung round them or hitched round the waist, all of the cheapest cotton cloth which through age and dirt had lost all colour and pattern. Each carried a *parang*, a sort of machete.

All morning they walked towards the looming mountains. Everyone was grim and serious now, beginning a long struggle for survival. There were no more jokes and no one sang. Each trudged quietly, deeply occupied in personal thoughts and problems.

Cicely's overwhelming feeling was again that she was neglecting her duty and abandoning her patients. She was conscious too of sensations of acute shock running through the whole party. They had all lost most of their possessions and, she felt, most of their self-respect. They had no idea what they were running away from or into. She knew that she was not the only one making tremendous efforts to be patient.

About midday they came to the last *kampong* before the mountain range. Most of the villagers were in the paddy fields, but those left behind came out and stared. They had never seen a white woman before. The shaggy pot-bellied children, some of them girls decked with small silver shields, also stared, not even realising that for Malay children the custom was to run screaming from white people. The villagers offered *rambulans* and sugar cane, and the party sat down for a rest. But within half an hour they were off again, and had left all other human life behind.

"It's so beautiful," said Cicely, looking at the contrast of mountains and jungle. "I find it hard to believe that we are still in Malaya. I associate the country so much with the monotony of rubber trees and surburban commonplaces."

The way now led upstream, and they walked up the river bed

because there was no path along the bank. They were often wading waist deep against the swift current, over boulders, through sinking sand and occasionally through thick jungle.

In the late afternoon they reached a gorge with a river running round a wide sandy beach on one bank. No. 1 party had camped there the previous night and had made some jungle huts into which they joyfully flung their loads before starting to collect firewood. After a consultation with Cobden Ramsey they decided that the evening rations would be rice, one *papaya* and a tin of pilchards. They bathed in the river and used banana leaves as plates. By the time it was dark they were ready for sleep. The carriers talked and laughed for two hours after the Europeans had become silent. The morale of the party had improved, and Cicely was conscious of a starry jungle night of dreams and the sound of running water.

Even with so little equipment, she thought, it was remarkable how long it took to do things, to unload, collect firewood and then leaves to make a bed, bathe, dry, share out the food, see to someone's leech bites and someone else's sore eye. Then a carrier wanted to turn back and she had to decide whether his troubles were due to malaria or to malingering. It was obvious that the man was an old chronic with considerable malnutrition.

In the morning they boiled rice and then set out again on the same sort of sticky upstream wading. At midday they passed No. 2 party's second camp by the waterside. At this point their path left the river and went straight up the hillside through deep jungle. It was slippery. Cicely often found herself climbing on all fours, and one of the worst problems were the leeches. The carriers cut little triangular sticks for everone so that they could flick the leeches off if they saw them in time. Cicely was constantly thankful that somehow she had blindly acquired the right kit for the journey. The tennis shoes were the best possible footwear, and the woolly stockings kept the sand out of her shoes and gave some protection from the leeches. The shirt and shorts were the best clothes for wading and for going through jungle. Every evening when they camped Ah Yong would park out her things in a barrier between them and the men. She would get out Cicely's sarong and send her off to bathe in the river. Then she would seize any of Cicely's clothes that she could find and wash them in the stream. When Cicely returned she would find Ah Yong crouching over the fire with the carriers, drying underclothes in sections.

It was hard going. The path was almost perpendicular, and none of them was well fed or in good training. For some time they travelled up a steep gorge, climbing huge boulders with the stream that was really only a slightly interrupted waterfall. Later the path became still steeper. Rain fell and the evening began to close in. In the deep jungle it was almost dark when they reached camp, which was to be the last camping site on the Trengganu side of the divide. It had none of the idyllic conditions of the night before. The camp was perched on a tiny space with not even a clearing and with everyone—trekkers, carriers and cooks—crowded together. There was a stream, but it was a mere trickle of water and offered little pleasure. It was also cold. Rain fell down the backs of their necks and it was almost impossible to cook the rice. The jungle huts were lightly built and not waterproof. They had also been built too short, so that all night the rain poured down on their feet. By now, like most of the others, Cicely had no dry garment.

For the first and only time she took the whisky from the medical supplies and handed it out with the dinner. They also opened the only tin of butter to eat with the rice. But when they tried to sleep they were all shivering with cold, and Cicely found little joy in piling on top of herself every garment she possessed in a sodden mass. Ah Yong opened her attaché case and produced a small dry towel from among her neatly folded possessions. This she put across her own and Cicely's necks, carefully arranging all the wet clothes, and then snuggled up, saying in Malay, "Amah very hot. Missee very cold. Very sorry."

Cicely knew that few of the party would be able to stand these conditions for long.

In the morning the rain still fell. Mist drifted through the trees and the whole of creation seemed dank and wretched. At dawn they coaxed up another fire for their rice and Bovril and filled their bottles with water. That day they were to cross the top of the mountain range and would not see a stream again until their evening camp. All their clothes were wet and they were a miserable crowd.

But as the day wore on things improved. There were signs of elephant and other game, and this cheered them. They were warmed by the steep climb through dense jungle. The sun banished the mist and drips. By midday they reached the top of the range. Even here trees grew too thickly to get much of a view. They halted for half an hour, drank water and ate a few biscuits. Cicely had to bandage Cobden Ramsey's feet. The canvas boots he had bought for the journey had been a poor investment. Falling to pieces, they had to be reinforced by elaborate bandaging on the outside.

They were now in the state of Pahang. The way lay steeply downhill. There was a path, but it was slippery, and Cicely's shoes were wearing out.

"I can see that I'm going to spend most of the afternoon walloping down on my behind," she said.

The Malay guide, who carried no load, went faster than the rest of the party could manage. It was always Cicely who called the halts. She did this deliberately because she noticed that if one of the men had to call a halt he immediately became irritable. But if she did it then everyone was pleased. She looked round frequently to see if anyone was falling too far behind, or if Cobden, who insisted on carrying his gun as well as an unwieldy load in a cricket bag on his shoulders, was turning blue.

"Have you noticed that we've seen no more leeches since we crossed the divide?" she said in a cheering tone. "I wonder why."

They heard the sound of running water for hours before they reached it. After an exasperating, slithering, bumping, mud-beplastered journey they reached another encampment beside a different river. Here there was only a narrow rocky strip between the jungle and the river bank, but there were huts and water, and they drank deeply and waded in to wash off the mud. Then they held a council to decide what to do next. The way was now downstream.

"If we push on hard," said Jerram, "we could probably get to the next camp tonight and so overtake No. 2 party."

"It seems to me," replied Cobden Ramsey thoughtfully, "that the advantages of overtaking the other party are few and the dangers of human friction are great. So let's have a nice easy afternoon."

There was general relief and smiles, and in contrast to the miserable camp of the night before they untied their packs in the early afternoon, spread out their belongings to dry and bathed at leisure in a decent, swirling river. One of the Malays went fishing, and in an extraordinarily short time he came back with half a dozen fish, at least eight inches long.

"I wish I'd seen how he did it," said Cicely, bubbling again for the first time in days.

They basked in the sun. They had time to push leaves into the rocky crannies for their sleeping place. Then, as the sun was leaving their gorge, they built big fires and stuck branches round them on which they hung their still damp garments. These made extraordinary leaping shadows until a shower of rain sent everyone scuttling out to grab them off the sticks. The rain doused the fires with hissing and spluttering.

They now felt that they had broken the back of the journey and so far all had gone well. The messages left by the previous parties written in the sand or pinned on the trees showed that they were getting on satisfactorily. Their food was lasting well and they had used few of their slender supply of tins.

Some of their anxieties were relieved, but they had others. Perhaps the most pressing of these was that no one knew what they were trekking to or surviving for.

Next morning there was more rain, but they were off in good time.

"I could almost dance with joy," said Cobden Ramsey, "because we're actually going to go downhill."

"Listen," said Jerram, about two hours later. "Voices. English voices."

They listened. Cicely could feel her heart pounding. It was at least partial success to hear English voices on the other side of the great mountain divide.

A tall bearded figure emerged through the jungle. Cicely recognised Fredericksen, a Dane on whose estate she had once stayed. With him was a forest officer and Brant, the leader of party No. 1. Fredericksen greeted her warmly and told her that he and the forest officer had escaped by Kuantan. But the rest of the news the men brought was all bad. They told them about the sinking of the *Prince of Wales* and the *Repulse*, about the Japanese advance and the British retreat from Kota Bahru.

"And the news from Trengganu?"

Brant shook his head sadly. "We've heard nothing," he said. "So I can't tell you anything about either Leslie Shield or the de Moubrays."

Now the going was quite pleasant. The stream gradually widened and became less wild and rough, with fewer fallen trees, and at midday it joined a wide river. On the opposite bank were two motorboats, a couple of small canoes and an attap shelter where men were cooking.

They were ferried across the deep water, and then the Malay forest rangers sat them down on the sand and gave them rice with roasted stink fish, coffee and bananas. They unpacked, paid off the carriers, and gave whatever tins they had left to the headman for the return journey, and climbed into the boats.

"We shall have to pack you in very carefully," said Brant. "The boats weren't built to take a party of this size." He made each person sit with his back against one side of the boat and his feet against the other, alternating the feet and backs.

The boats were swift, powerful and skilfully manned. Cicely found the river beautiful and enjoyed the way their craft cut through the water. At some of the rapids they had to get out and walk, but generally only the men were turned out and Ah Yong and Cicely were left in the boats as passengers. It was Cicely's first and only experience of shooting rapids, and she enjoyed it immensely.

Three days later they reached their objective, the railway

halt at Tembeling. They paid the boatmen, put the luggage on to a bullock cart with Ah Yong on top to look after it, and walked a mile to the railway station through the gathering darkness.

The place had already been bombed, and thousands of refugees from Kelantan, Trengganu and Pahang had already passed through. More were huddled on the platform. There was a curious atmosphere of tension, patience, fatalism and indifference which Cicely had never encountered before. She soon came to realise that this goes with war. Chinese, Malays, Tamils and Europeans were all the same. When the little local train drew in it was blacked out. Everyone climbed in quietly and sat huddled where they could. Other Europeans were in Cicely's carriage, and they began to swap stories, but without much interest and only to pass the time. They travelled north to Kuala Lipis, where they arrived late at night and in pouring rain.

Cicely was given a two-bedded hospital room to share with Ah Yong. She lay luxuriously in a bath, soaking the grime from her skin and the stiffness from her joints. When she returned to the bedroom the Chinese woman looked pleased.

"Why, Ah Yong," cried Cicely. "What a wonderful surprise! However did you manage it?"

To her astonishment, laid out ready on the bed was her satin nightgown, and on the dressing-table were the shagreen and silver mirror and the little West African leather box. When she threw them away on the other side of the mountain Ah Yong had rescued them and carried them packed in her attaché case with her own belongings.

All next day, Cicely sat in the train with her feet up on a haversack, contemplating her swollen ankles and listening to horror stories about the Japanese invasion. These stories, she decided, lost nothing in the telling. In the carriage were two young Australian soldiers who drank beer all the way and kept asserting that nothing on earth would make them fight. Looking at them, Cicely could not help feeling that it was a sinister augury for the future.

CHAPTER VIII

SINGAPORE, THE IMPREGNABLE fortress, 20 December, 1941. Cicely felt safe at last. She walked from the train on her painful feet, carrying her few remaining possessions in a small sack.

On the platform was Dr MacGregor, the Director of Medical Services, bluff and tactless. He shook hands.

"All you doctors running away from your jobs up country. I don't know what to do with you all in Singapore."

Thoughts of the patients abandoned in Kuala Trengganu brought back her pain. But she jerked her mind away and remembered her new job. If there were too many doctors in Singapore she would go to India immediately.

Next morning she went to say this to Dr MacGregor. But his first remark was, "You can look after all the bombed and blasted babies."

"What do you mean?" asked Cicely uncertainly.

"Singapore has been bombed," he said. "There's a lot of damage in the Chinese quarters, and thousands of children are wounded or lost."

"What do you want me to do?"

"Your job," he told her, "is to empty the children's wards in Singapore General Hospital to provide more room for casualties from the bombing. You must also make arrangements for the lost and homeless children. You can have a car and start right away."

"It's amazing what you can get used to," Cicely said a few days later to Edith Zehnder, a member of the lay committee which was helping with the lost children.

She was already deeply involved in her work, driving all over Singapore, trying to do a thousand different things and developing an arduous routine, often with bombs dropping round her.

"It's not only a question of getting used to it," said Mrs Zehnder. "None of us can really face the thinking. It's easier just to get on with the job."

It was true. No one wanted to think. But sometimes reality was forced into Cicely's mind.

One day she was in the doctors' mess in the hospital eating a quick meal before hurrying to a children's Home. Other doctors were chatting, mostly about patients and living conditions. No one talked much about the war.

"It could be a rare form of beri-beri."

"Do you think . . .?"

The door opened suddenly and the question was left unasked. A frightened Eurasian nurse rushed in and screamed, "They've crossed the Slim river. They're nearly here." She began to sob loudly.

For weeks the general belief had been that the Japanese were being allowed to advance quickly down the peninsula because the Allies were going to defend the Slim. This river had become for them all a symbol of the resistance.

There was a queasy silence. Then one of the doctors burst out.

"We've been deceived with a million lies just to suit Bumbledom's convenience. Singapore is supposed to be a fortress but it bloody well isn't. Millions of pounds have been wasted on building the naval base, yet it's on the north side of the island, only a thousand yards from the Johore mainland. How in Heaven's name is that going to help us? It'll be Johore next. Then over the Straits. Impregnable fortress my eye."

But Cicely, like most of the others, still could not really take it in. She left the room silently. Getting on with her work seemed the only thing to do.

Air raids, as well as living conditions, were worse each day. She moved into the General Hospital to give what help she could with the wounded. In the evenings, after her long day's work, she was there to help with casualties, do surgical operations and give anaesthetics.

A few days later, in the middle of her ward round, there was a sudden noise so loud that several nurses dived under beds. They soon realised with a shock that they were being shelled.

The thought that the Japanese now had guns on the mainland big enough and near enough to hit them was unbearable. In the doctors' mess the atmosphere was grim, and someone said, "I'm sure we'll get reinforcements."

There was some relief. Cicely realised that everyone longed to believe this, and so hope was still in the air.

On 31 January they heard that the Allies had withdrawn from the mainland to Singapore Island.

"Johore is being evacuated and the Causeway is being blown up."

"Well," Cicely said calmly, surprised at her own steadiness, "we're going to share with Malta the distinction of being a besieged island."

But the destruction of the Causeway did not prevent the Japanese from landing on the Island.

Next day the Director of Medical Services gave instructions that the children in the General Hospital were to be moved to Cicely's section of Tan Tock Seng, because the whole of the General Hospital was needed for casualties. Cicely's nightmare began.

"Not the best place to protect sick children," said Cicely ruefully.

She paused for a moment in the job of helping the ambulance drivers unload the hundred children. She knew that there would also be forty from St Andrew's Orthopaedic Hospital. These were children in plaster frames, many with tuberculous spines.

"Look at the buildings!" she said despairingly to Dr Margaret Smallwood, who had been sent to help her. "Just fragile bungalows with no protection against blast or bombs, and they're not even blacked out."

"And there's no hot water and nowhere to cook," said Dr Smallwood.

Cicely was the only doctor sleeping in the children's section. This meant that she could hardly ever go to bed. There were frequent emergencies among her own babies, and new patients arrived by ambulance all the time.

Each day the shelling was heavier. The hospital staff gradually disappeared, usually without warning. Food and water were scarce. Cicely knew that none of them could last long under these conditions.

One night, as on most nights, she was called to the Admissions Ward. By now she was so tired that it was difficult even to remain upright, and she was only dimly aware that the shelling was heavier than usual. She did not notice Bertha Wong, a Chinese nurse who had come from St Andrew's Hospital with the orthopaedic children. Nurse Wong spoke to Cicely in her comforting sing-song voice.

"You again, Dr Williams, always you."

Cicely raised her head and smiled.

"And always you, Miss Wong," she said, returning the compliment. Bertha Wong had never failed to come on duty, and she gave Cicely a secure feeling that she never would fail.

A newly arrived child, a baby of about a year old, lay disconcertingly still. Cicely's diagnosis was swift.

"Oh God," she said, "diphtheria. As if we didn't have enough troubles already! I daren't take it in. It'll have to go to the Fever Hospital. Is the ambulance still there, by any chance?"

"No, Doctor, it drove off straight away."

"Damn. I'll have to take it there myself."

"But the shelling, Doctor, it's terrible outside. The danger. You may be killed."

"I daren't admit a case of diphtheria. Don't worry, nurse. The Middleton Hospital is only a few hundred yards away."

She picked up the sick child and pushed herself out through the swing doors and into the eerie, flashing night.

In twenty minutes she was back on the ward, stronger now and ready for the night's work.

The sight of the children forced back into her mind the sorrow and fear that fatigue and activity had kept at bay. There were more sick babies than she could count, and they all needed more food and medical attention than anyone could give them.

"And there's no time to give them any love at all." Row upon row of quiet, scared little faces peered through cot bars.

For night duty there was now only one amah in a ward for sixty children, and she threw up her hands, said, "I can't bear it," and rushed away.

Cicely spent the rest of the night looking after the ward. Some of the children, especially those who had been wounded previously, had screaming horrors during the shelling and bombing. She collected the worst ones at one end and went constantly from one to the other. Outside the fighting was continuous. It seemed to Cicely that they were in the middle of a non-stop battle with guns infiltrating all round the hospital.

Among the children with screaming terrors there was one piece of comic relief. A little Malay boy, Awong, had been in Singapore General Hospital for sixteen months. He had now nearly recovered and was about two years old. Whenever the noise of bombardment subsided Cicely could hear from his cot a soft, "Wisha, wisha, wisha, wisha, bang!", a perfect imitation of the shell. Or "Bow wow, wow, wow," when the dogs had been barking.

"It's amazing how that child lacks fear," said Bertha Wong, who had slipped into the ward for a few minutes.

"I am afraid it's only an illustration of the confidence of the 'protected' child," answered Cicely. "Unlike many of the other children who have had grim experiences, he simply doesn't know what it's all about."

By morning, Friday the 13th, she had been working for twenty-four hours continuously. But most of the day staff failed to turn up, among them Doctor Heng, the house physician. Instead of going to bed she would now have to work through another busy day.

Sudden rage and hopelessness swept over her, and she burst

out to Bertha Wong, "It's disgraceful that we've heard nothing from headquarters about the European women being evacuated. It's typical of things here in Malaya that more attention is paid to equipment than to people. The Q.A.A.N.S. have gone. Why should the rest stay behind?"

"If you go, all the nurses will leave," said Bertha Wong, quietly.

"They're leaving anyway," retorted Cicely. "You are one of the few still on duty, Nurse Wong."

She rang up Doctor Bowyer, the Chief Medical Officer of the General Hospital, and told him that she thought the women ought to leave. His reply was like a knell.

"It's too late, Cicely. The last ship has gone."

Friday night was even worse, and the amah in the older children's ward brought all her family of thirteen people to live in a room about ten feet square next to the ward. In desperate need of more helping hands, Cicely went to this room and threatened to turn out anyone of a size to work who did not do so. In this way the amah's old father and her two children were soon helping to wash the clothes and sweep the floor.

At seven o'clock the day staff went off duty. Cicely said she would look after the babies' wards for an hour until the night staff arrived. But only Bertha Wong came, although the doctors were living 200 yards away. The road was under fire and the soldiers barred their way.

All night Cicely toured the wards, doing what she could, knowing how much more was needed. The shelling was the heaviest ever, and even the most placid babies and the sickest children were upset.

In the early hours bits of metal started to fly round the ward.

"I think this is the end," said Cicely to herself. It felt like the end of the world. She picked up the babies in armfuls and put them under beds, on which she piled three or four mattresses. Some cried and struggled. Some whimpered. Some were floppy like toys. One was sick over her. She ran backwards and forwards from one group to the next, comforting, tending, occasionally even treating.

"Who are those men?" she asked, nor really caring. It was dawn, and she suddenly realised that the firing had ceased. But there was no one to answer. The men were wounded British soldiers, and Cicely tended them. It was now two days since she had slept.

The day staff arrived at 7 a.m., punctually and almost briskly. Cicely went off duty and lay down under her bed, too tired even to shift the pillow.

Soon a voice called her.

"Doctor Williams. Doctor Williams."

She wasn't even properly asleep. It couldn't have been more than five minutes since she lay down. Dr Margaret Smallwood was standing over her.

"We have orders to evacuate the hospital in twelve minutes. The ambulances are already arriving. The Bishop* himself has come with some people to help us shift the children."

She jumped up, quickly finding reserves of strength, and hurried across the courtyard. The Bishop and his volunteers, among them Miss Simmonds, were already helping the nurses and ambulance men to load the children into the ambulances.

"Everything is becoming disintegrated, including standards," said Miss Simmonds, who was just as efficient and energetic in the existing chaos as she had been when she was organising the rural health services. "Look at those soldiers." Across the street a group of Australians looked disorganised and defeated, and were looting the shops. Farther down the road others had thrown away their equipment and sat in rows with their boots off. "These deserting soldiers are terrible," she continued. "They're pushing women and children out of the way, and trampling on them to protect themselves from the bombs."

"I'm finding it difficult to drive because of the holes in the roads," said Cicely. Rubbish and rubble lay everywhere in gigantic piles. Tangled masses of wires, electric, telephone and telegraph, were strewn across the street, with smashed cars, trucks, trams and buses. Shops were shuttered and deserted. Bombs were still falling, and rescuers were digging in the rubble.

* John Wilson, Bishop of Singapore, now Bishop of Birmingham.

"Hundreds of Chinese civilians are still in their homes, just waiting to die," said Miss Simmonds.

"He told me to take them to Outram Road Jail. God knows what we shall find."

As soon as they arrived at the jail the two women set to work to sweep out an old storeroom before the ambulances arrived.

"There's a tap in the courtyard."

"That's something to be thankful for. But there's no water inside the building."

Cicely left Miss Simmonds at the jail, as well as Ah Yong, who had come to help her soon after their journey over the mountains, and went back to the General Hospital.

"The orders have been changed, Dr Williams," a nurse told her. "The babies are to stay here."

"Where are they?" asked Cicely, alarmed.

"In the Dental Department. We've just finished putting them there."

"But there aren't any beds in the Dental Department."

"All the same, Doctor, that's where they are."

Cicely hurried upstairs. In the Dental Department she saw her children and the floor and that was all. There was everything to do, no one to do it and nothing to do it with.

She went to the kitchen and asked for food for her babies. The man in charge of the stores looked unhelpful and said they couldn't cook for any more people.

Cicely knew that he was justified. The General Hospital was supposed to have a thousand beds, but that day it contained at least 10,000 people. Everyone seemed to be sheltering there—civilians, deserting soldiers and anybody who felt that the hospital might be some protection. All the same, the man's uninvolved refusal annoyed her.

In the store she found an administrative officer. He gave her a bag of rice, some tins, including dried milk, and coal pots with two sacks of charcoal. He told her that they would have to cook the food themselves.

"But where can we cook?" said Bertha Wong. "We can't put coal pots on the verandah because metal is flying about."

"We'll have to light fires indoors," said Cicely. "I shall boil the milk on the bunsen burners in the Dental Department."

While she was cooking the rice three amahs came from St Andrew's Hospital to help, but they looked at the children, said they were too dirty, and went away.

"I'm going to drive back to Tan Tock Seng and fetch those two nurses who were left behind," said Cicely.

"But, Doctor," said Nurse Wong in alarm, "there is a raid. The bombs are falling. Please go later."

"No," said Cicely. "We can't go on like this much longer. The babies will die if they are not nursed, and downstairs in Casualty there are hundreds of wounded waiting for attention."

At eight o'clock that evening more nurses arrived, and Cicely felt that she could now go back to the Jail. She was now so tired that she could scarcely stand and scarcely see. She curled up on the floor and found the noise of shells overhead almost pleasant. The prison walls felt so secure after the babies' wards in Tan Tock Seng.

They couldn't find any lavatories in the jail. "And it's odd," Cicely remarked to Miss Simmonds, "how we don't seem to need them." It was not the only time that she experienced conditions in which the body can more or less stop eating, drinking, excreting and sleeping for long periods of time.

But not the children. The next day was Sunday, and Cicely spent it in the Dental Department in the hopeless task of trying to care for the children.

Meanwhile Japanese planes flew over in couples, dropping bombs and machine-gunning.

"Our anti-aircraft guns now seem too exhausted to hit them," said Cicely to Dr Smallwood. There was shelling and gunfire all day, and sniping even inside the hospital grounds. In the middle of it all the hospital water supply failed.

"This is the end," said Cicely. "How can the children survive this?"

Conditions inside the hospital were deteriorating. Part of the building had been hit. The lower storeys were filled with housands of peop le jostling, moving aimlessly, sitting or lying.

There were patients in the wards and corridors, on beds, chairs or floors. Dead bodies were piled at intervals in the corridors. Among them wandered nurses, orderlies, coolies, their relatives, and also some Army deserters, British, Australian and Indian, taking shelter, doing no work, grabbing the food and trampling on the helpless. In the midst of it all some people continued to do their jobs, caring for casualties, working the operating theatres and X-ray rooms. And all the time the ambulances continued to arrive with their loads.

Maud Pereira, a Health Nurse, offered to look after the children's wards with the aid of her family. Cicely began to think of sleep.

"I'm going to sleep on the floor of the Dental Museum because it's near the children," she announced, knowing that she would probably be alone up there with Miss Simmonds, for no one else would want to sleep on the top storey.

Blackout in the museum was rudimentary, and she crawled through darkness. Shells were still coming over, but she managed to doze. Suddenly the museum was filled with light, and Tratman, the Professor of Dentistry, was framed in the doorway. He spoke in a strange, deliberate voice.

"You can put on the lights. There's an armistice."

The words took time to penetrate Cicely's mind. "Why?" she said, tensely. "Who has given in?"

"We have," said the Professor.

Next morning there was still no water. Several of Cicely's babies had died in the night, and their bodies were piled in a corner. Bishop Wilson arrived in his car, and when he saw what was happening he drove away and fetched five A.R.P. tins of water from St Andrew's Hospital.

Later that morning Cicely was interrupted in her work by a sister who whispered, "The Director of Medical Services has arrived."

Startled, Cicely walked down the ward to greet him, but he took no notice. He was looking at the children.

"Even Sepoy Lines is better than this," he said. "I'll arrange it."

Sepoy Lines was a maternity hospital a few hundred yards away.

"But that was evacuated three days ago because it was so badly shelled," said Cicely anxiously.

"It's still better than this."

She submitted, feeling doubtful and desperate. Not trusting herself to wait peacefully for the ambulances she drove to Mount Sophia to see a brood of about a hundred lost children at Nam Wah. She saw that these children, under the care of a practical woman called Mrs Loveridge, were doing much better than her own babies. Mrs Loveridge had refused to move, and so had managed to keep together most of her staff, food and equipment, all of which Cicely had now virtually lost.

"You make me realise," she said, "that shifting from place to place as we have done is a sort of disease that people get in war time, and is one of its worst horrors."

No one tried to stop her in the streets. On the way home she saw Japanese soldiers for the first time. They were walking about in small batches, looking pleased. She even saw some of them trying to stop the looting.

"But there isn't any water after all," cried Cicely, dismayed. "We can't look after sick babies here."

She went back to the General Hospital with two of the nurses to fetch water in cans. Eventually someone sent a water cart with the explanation that it had been forgotten.

"That's typical of the whole situation," she groaned. "People tell you to go somewhere and then don't send you the stuff you need. You go and then wish you hadn't."

But somehow they managed to wash and feed the children. Occasionally there was even some gas. Otherwise they used their coal pots and charcoal. Meanwhile disorganised people from outside wandered in and out, looting vaguely and sometimes taking the food off the fire. Once Cicely got hold of three disreputable and defeated British soldiers and made them guard her pots while she scrubbed floors, sluiced latrines and washed babies. Then she made them tea in payment.

The Japanese soldiers also wandered in and out and were objects of interest and fear.

"There's something simian about them," said Cicely. "They're inquisitive like monkeys."

By the following evening most of her children were fed and in bed, and there were sheets and towels, gas, water and food. But it did not last. Aston, the hospital secretary who had given her food for the babies in the General Hospital, came to the ward. Cicely could see at once that he brought bad news.

"I'm sorry, Doctor Williams. You've all got to move again."

"Oh no." Agreement was unbearable.

"The Japanese are taking over all these hospitals for their own casualties. Our patients are to go to the Mental Hospital." The Japanese had renamed this hospital *Myako* meaning victory. The mental hospital patients had already been transferred to a hospital on one of the islands.

Moving again was almost more than Cicely could bear, but she tried to control her feelings through activity. During the afternoon two of the babies died. She paused in her work and said, "I'm going to take the bodies to the pit."

She referred to a hole in the grounds of the General Hospital. It had been a big excavation started by the Public Works Department to make a water tank, but was now used as a large communal grave.

It was already half-full and decomposing. She dropped the two little bodies in as gently as possible and turned away, heaving.

Many of the children left in the wards were seriously ill. She greatly feared what would await them in the Mental Hospital.

"A lady and gentleman have come to see you, Doctor Williams."

A worried nurse hurried to Cicely, who was making a pile of blankets in a corner of the ward, ready to move them into the ambulances when the Japanese weren't looking. They had given orders that no equipment was to be taken with the children. She looked up and saw a neatly dressed Chinese couple in the far corner. The woman carried a tin of baby food and a feeding bottle.

"They have come for their baby, Doctor, but we cannot find it. We have searched all the hospital and it is nowhere."

Cicely's heart jerked. All the children's bed tickets had been lost in the last move, and there was no means of identifying either those who had died or those who were too young to know who they were.

"Perhaps it has died."

"Perhaps, Doctor." The nurse stood looking at her feet.

"All right," said Cicely. "I had better see the parents."

An idea flashed and exploded in her brain, stripped off layers of habit, and left a new stark outline.

She had about ten seconds to decide, the time it took to walk down the ward. On either side the babies lay in rows, sick, dying, abandoned and now nameless. Surely, she felt, we can do something. If we go on like this they will soon all be dead. Hopeless situations demand new remedies, unrelated to customary solutions.

Waiting at the end of the ward stood the parents of the lost baby. The mother's face was unmoving. Emotion showed only in her forefinger drumming against the feeding bottle.

"I am sorry to tell you," said Cicely, keeping her voice steady, "your baby has died."

The quiet Chinese faces were inscrutable. Cicely paused, gulped, and then spoke out from deep inside her.

"*You can have another baby if you would like to choose one.*"

There was a pause, and an atmosphere of surprise as everyone took in what she had said. Then big smiles broke on both the parents' faces. They went up to a jolly little Chinese two-year-old, who made friends immediately. In five minutes all three had gone, before Cicely had had time to absorb what she had done.

As they left the ward the mother turned to Cicely.

"You are giving away the babies, then? Is that right?"

"Yes," said Cicely, and her voice seemed to have sunk to a

deep bass. "Yes, that's right. We are giving away the babies," and she added, more to herself or to God than to the Chinese, "I do now believe that virtually any sort of home will probably be better for these children than anything that we can do for them."

The word soon went round. Another couple came, and soon afterwards others. They had all heard that the doctors were "giving away children for nothing." Altogether Cicely "gave away" ten that morning. She tried to arrange these adoptions as well as possible, but in her heart she knew that this was nothing but a little balm to her own conscience. She found it extraordinary to watch the commercial way in which some of the Chinese examined these children, and the care with which they inspected the genitals before risking an adoption. One mother, whose baby had died, was genuinely delighted to get another. But another, recognising her own child, said, "No, I won't take him. He's too thin. I don't want him back."

"Come," said Cicely. "I need your help."

The young medical orderly looked defeated, but roused himself to co-operate. A voluntary helper had also been sent to help with the move.

"When we have loaded the ambulances please sit beside me in the car in case of trouble."

Together the remaining staff had looted the Maternity Hospital for mackintosh sheets, blankets, cots, mattresses, linen and cooking utensils. They took pots of rice and tins of water, cooking pots and charcoal stoves, loaded the ambulances and started the slow ten-mile journey to the Mental Hospital.

"The Japanese seem to be having a bit of a parade in the town," Cicely said to her young companion. At frequent intervals the convoy of ambulances was held up by tanks and troops.

"Look out!" he cried, suddenly alert, as a Japanese officer backed his car straight into Cicely's. There was a horrid pause, then a crash much louder than the impact seemed to warrant.

"Oh God," groaned Cicely. "What now?"

The Japanese climbed out of his car and walked towards them, angry and menacing. She gripped the steering wheel, terrified, not daring to move. But all he did was bellow "Yah," climb back into his car and drive away quickly.

At the Mental Hospital there was a queue of ambulances, and they could not get within 200 yards of their wards. There were no trolleys or people to help unload the patients.

"We shall have to do it ourselves," said Cicely, trying not to think about her painful, swollen feet. Months and years later, when she had been through much worse experiences, she still felt the pain in her feet when she remembered moving all those children in plasters, and the hundreds of wretched people being transferred from other hospitals.

The doctors, nurses and voluntary helpers became exhausted carrying the stretchers. When they could work no longer they had to leave patients lying in the corridors until someone had the energy to move them. Even when they reached the ward there was only the floor: no beds, no water, no food.

Cicely and her staff gave the children milk and the boiled rice. But no one else had brought any food, although six hundred patients had been moved into the hospital that day. Cicely's bag of rice had to provide a meal for everyone. All night the patients lay on bare concrete in the wards and cried for water.

Again Maud Pereira and her family took over for the night. Cicely and Miss Bryant, a matron at one of the hospitals, were taken to a small house where doctors and nurses were sleeping. About a hundred exhausted people were lying on the floor in every room and corridor. The two women had brought a mattress. They dropped it on the floor of a passage and fell asleep immediately.

She was woken by the stink from her own clothes. When they carried the children into the Mental Hospital many of them had been in the ambulances for six hours and were filthy. Cicely now found she could only sleep after she had taken off her dress and hung it out of the window. She was restless until morning about her babies and listening to the noise made by the hundred sleeping people round her. After the first night she took up quarters with Ah Yong in a room at the end of the children's ward.

Cicely's main problem now was how to get the work done. Miss Bryant suggested that the older children should help. Like everyone else, she was showing signs of strain. Cicely admired the way she never flagged, and was always efficient and methodical.

"None of them is really well enough," said Cicely, doubtfully.

"There's a boy called Sockalingnam in the schoolboys' ward. Nurse Benjamin has been training him to look after the other children. Then there's Matthew."

"But he has a T.B. hip."

"He's practically recovered now."

"All the same," said Cicely, "he still needs many months of rest."

"Can you suggest what else we do?" Miss Bryant's voice contained a faint edge of irony.

"Yes," said Cicely angrily. "Choose some of these parasitic Europeans. There are dozens of them sitting about and doing nothing."

"Useless," said Miss Bryant. "Those who are mentally capable of it are working hard. We won't get anywhere with the others, nor with the Mental Hospital's amahs. They're dreadful. They do no work and steal everything they can lay their hands on. Matthew is worth dozens of them."

Cicely felt unhappy but agreed to use Matthew, knowing that it might cripple him for life. The child had the same dogged enthusiasm as those who had cared for him. During the next few weeks he worked as hard on the ward as Cicely herself, and only stopped when his hip trouble broke out again, this time incurably.

One day a familiar figure appeared in the ward.

"Jack," cried Cicely, delighted. It was Jack Monro, the professor of surgery. "Have you come to help?"

"Well, sort of." He grinned, gave a small embarrassed cough and said, "Could I borrow one of those things for a while?"

"Borrow a baby? Why on earth . . .?"

He laughed. "No, not a baby. A cot. I need an instrument trolley, and a cot is about the next best thing."

"But my babies need the cots."

"I need one too, for an instrument trolley."

She gave way. "All right. Take your damned cot. But you are deeply in my debt for it."

"Of course." He gave her an affectionate smile and walked to the nearest cot. He lifted out the child, together with the mattress, swung it in the air to make it laugh, laid it tenderly on the floor and walked off down the corridor trundling the empty rattling cot behind him.

She soon forgave him. He installed himself in the hospital and organised not only the many necessary surgical operations but also the water supply, drainage and food. He even managed to find some orderlies.

After a few days conditions were improving, and she decided to try to recover her possessions from Tan Tock Seng, which was now in the hands of the Japanese.

She drove to the local Japanese High Command. No one tried to stop her except a Japanese soldier who seemed to want the car. She argued fiercely. He did not persist, and wandered away aimlessly.

She passed a procession of Europeans being marched from Raffles Hotel to internment in Katong. They were mostly family groups, with mothers and fathers carrying children and dragging their luggage as best they could.

In the Japanese Headquarters everything was amazingly easy. A soldier sitting at a desk behind the door spoke enough English to communicate, and she returned to her car with a note written in Japanese which apparently authorised her to go back to Tan Tock Seng to collect her possessions.

But 100 yards further on the car spluttered and ran out of petrol. No more was available. She had no alternative but to return to the Myako.

"I don't see how I can get back to Tan Tock Seng now," said Cicely sadly to Professor Monro. "I suppose all my belongings will be lost, all for the want of a few teaspoons of petrol."

"I'd better introduce you to Bert and Des," he answered.

"Bert and Des?"

"Two Australian soldiers who are pals of mine. They've put Red Cross Bands on their hats. They have a lorry and they bring food supplies to the hospital. God knows why. No one told them to do it. I'll introduce them."

"Sure," said Bert, large, redfaced and purposeful. "I'll take you to Tan Tock Seng. Just hop in."

Des looked like a weasel and was rather silent. He gave Cicely the impression that he noticed details.

She sat between them in the front of the "ambulance", an old green van with red crosses painted on the sides. They drove in silence across the island. All around lay derelict planes, cars, smashed lorries and the remains of disasters.

"Better do some milking," said Bert to Des at last.

Cicely looked round for a cow.

"Looks fresh, that one," said Des, jerking his head at a crashed lorry on which the rust had not yet settled.

"Pass the pipe."

Bert halted, and Des scuttled across the road with a tube and can and sucked out the petrol tank.

"That's how we keep going," said Bert. "Have to keep a lookout for fresh smashes. The Nips don't provide the juice, only permits." He laughed and waved a large red card at her, written in both Japanese and English. It certified that the bearer was acting on behalf of the Transport Department of the hospital.

"Phoney, of course," laughed Bert. "But it gets us through."

The guard at the gate of the Cold Storage Company glanced at the card and ran to open the big wire gates.

"See," said Bert with a grin. "They accept it."

They parked at the back and led her inside, where they all sat down at a small table with a clean check cloth. To Cicely's astonishment a Malay boy appeared and gave them an excellent breakfast of Dover sole, the last she was to see for years. After breakfast they filled their ambulance with frozen meat and other supplies to take back to the Mental Hospital, and on the way they called at Tan Tock Seng.

"Like me to come in with you?" asked Bert.

But she wanted to be alone when she first saw her precious possessions again.

"I'll be here if you want me," said Bert, understandingly.

Her room had been looted and her books scattered. She managed to save the Oxford Book of English Verse and the copy of Horace which her father had given her. At the back of a shelf she found the paper on rickets which she had carefully carried on her back out of Trengganu. She felt pleased that this was not lost to posterity, and then relieved that she could still feel pleased.

On the way back she was conscious of increasing pain and nausea in waves.

"You feeling all right?" asked Bert.

"It must be the fumes from the engine. I'll lie down when I get back."

But when they arrived at the hospital she heard that an urgent doctors' meeting was already in progress. Jack Monro was in the chair.

"The question is," he said as she came in, "are we willing to go on working under Asiatic doctors or do we prefer internment? The Japanese have given us the choice."

"I choose work," said Cicely. "How can we choose internment when there is so much to do?"

There were murmurs of approval and the decision was almost unanimous.

"I'm glad you feel like that," said Jack Monro.

She soon realised that she was suffering from dysentery. The disease was all over the hospital. During the next few days she became increasingly thankful to retire at intervals to the mattress on the floor in the room which she shared with Ah Yong.

Then the order came that she was to be interned, but by this time she was so ill that it scarcely affected her. She felt only thankful because she knew that she could no longer work. She gave most of her remaining possessions to the nurses and to Ah Yong. She asked the hospital authorities to keep Ah Yong on as an amah, but she never saw her again.

The next few weeks were terrible to those of sound mind and body, but they left little impression on Cicely. She was now severely ill, and knew that her life was in danger. Nightmares, both sleeping and waking, ebbed and flowed through her mind, and the mixture of fantasy and reality increased the chaos of memories.

The day she was interned she could still walk. A week before this, at ten o'clock on a Tuesday morning, she and many hundreds of other Europeans had collected in the *padang** in front of the municipal building. They stood in the hot sun for several hours without either food or water while the Japanese moved up and down the lines questioning those they chose. In the end the Japanese authorities decided to intern about 2,000 European men and 300 women and children. They were lined up and marched from the *padang* to some houses in Katong about five miles away. There were a few cars and lorries for the very young, for the decrepit and for some of the luggage. They had been told to bring only what they could carry, and they were advised to bring "clothing for ten days". Afterwards they were told that this should have been "food for ten days".

In Katong the women and children were sent to two large houses, one of which had belonged to the Sultan of Trengganu. Each house contained only household furniture, and the only lavatories were two commodes. No food was provided for twenty-four hours, but after that a few of the internees were allowed to go out and collect some. The women had to do all the work, including burying the night soil in the garden, where wired-off spaces indicated the suspected presence of land mines. The Japanese provided no beds, no utensils, no food and no assistance. Each day the number of internees increased. By the time Cicely was ordered to leave the hospital and

* Field.

go into internment there was considerable overcrowding. She shared a room with several other people. She still had her mattress and she clung to it. Soon she could not leave it. Her dysentery was getting worse. She knew that she was a danger to everyone, and she announced that she thought it would be better if she was moved back to the Mental Hospital. Somehow arrangements were made, but not before she was incontinent and nearly unconscious. She vaguely remembered being carried down the stairs on a stretcher and pushed into an ambulance, where she fainted again. She half-woke to find someone bending over her and taking her pulse. A voice said, "I just wanted to make certain that I wasn't carrying a corpse."

She felt she was floating on a shining orange cloud with a loud and hideous hum enveloping her head. She could feel her stomach heaving and her tired muscles too weak to respond. I'm dead, she thought, I'm already dead.

She came to on the floor of the Myako Hospital and found that she could just crawl to the latrines, which were three open pits out on the verandah. Men and women, sick and wounded, were mixed up and lying along the walls. Later she realised that everything was chaotic because the nursing sisters had been interned and the Chinese nurses were disorganised.

A few hours after she arrived Professor Monro found her. He managed to collect for her a bed, a spoon, a cup and a bowl. This felt like luxury, and after a few days she began to improve and even to appreciate not having to stand on her feet. All around her internees were suffering from dysentery and wounds, but she improved steadily. She never knew how long she spent in the Myako, but it seemed like a blessed pause in the disorganised life that had been going on since the beginning of November. She had just reached the stage when she could walk out of the ward and on to the verandah when orders came that she was to go back to camp immediately. The Japanese had brought in a new batch of bad cases of dysentery, and more space was needed.

CHAPTER IX

So SHE WENT back to prison, but not to Katong because while she was ill the second great march had taken place and all the internees had been moved into Changi Prison, which lay conspicuously on the eastern end of the island, about two miles from the sea.

Still weak on her legs, she climbed down from the back of the lorry and tottered through the big iron gates, which clanged behind her. Concrete walls loomed ahead. Women were queuing in the courtyard. They glanced round with curious expressions on their faces, half-furtive, half-frightened. Later Cicely realised that these attitudes were part of prison life and unavoidable, persisting not only during captivity but for years afterwards. The experienced can diagnose a jailbird across a room.

A woman left the queue and came forward. Cicely recognised Patricia Elliott, the doctor from the Anglican Mission Hospital. She greeted Cicely warmly and told her as much as she knew of what was going on.

"Life isn't easy," she said, "but the internees are fairly civilised."

"Are we allowed to visit the men?" asked Cicely. She was wondering about medical facilities. Among the six women doctors only she and Dr Elliott were specialists, and none of them were surgeons. Her friend, Jack Monro, the professor of surgery, was a prisoner on the men's side.

"Officially no," said Dr Elliott. "The Japanese are taking trouble to make sure there's no communication. But some enterprising souls have already solved the problem by going over the roofs and also, I'm told, through the drains."

Cicely laughed.

"Come and see round the place," said Patricia Elliott,

sweeping her arm in mock hospitality. "I'll give you a conducted tour. As you are probably aware, Changi was a civilian jail and supposed to be fairly modern. But where it isn't actually falling down it lets in the rain."

"Are you overcrowded?"

"Not really. At the moment we have space to move and breathe, but I don't know how long it will last. The Japanese bring in more people every day."

By the time they left Changi three years later their numbers had increased very seriously.

The jail was divided into large concrete blocks of buildings with about forty cells on each of five storeys. The cells opened on to gangways with iron railings. Each cell was about 8 feet by 12 feet with a small barred window high up in the wall, a concrete platform in the middle for sleeping, and a lavatory in the corner.

"We call those the 'squatters'," said Dr Elliott, "and the cell itself is a 'bed-squatter'."

There were only a couple of bathrooms in the whole building. Everyone had to wash as best they could in the cells or under the row of showers in the courtyard, which were turned on for half-an-hour morning and evening.

"We've kept this bed-squatter for you," said Dr Elliott. "It's bleak, but you'll get used to it."

Cicely felt grateful. At least she had somewhere of her own, and after her experiences in recent weeks this seemed luxurious.

"How about the food?"

"We don't get much," said Dr Elliott, "and cooking is an enormous problem. The trouble is that all the prison kitchens are on the men's side, yet the Japanese have ordered us to do our own cooking here on the women's side."

"How do you manage?"

"They have supplied a few cooking pots and put some tarpaulin sheets against the wall, but tarpaulin's no good against tropical rain and we only have a few amateur women to do the cooking."

Here Dr Elliott looked embarrassed and obviously wanted to get something off her chest.

"Actually, Cicely, we thought you might look after the food. We formed a medical committee of all the women doctors, and provisionally we have appointed you as dietician. Subject to your consent, of course." She looked slightly wistful.

"Dietician? But I'm a children's specialist." Cicely did not conceal her disappointment.

"I know. But you weren't here and Margaret Smallwood has organised the children. She's doing a magnificent job of work and sees every child every day. It's helping the mothers enormously."

"Wonderful," said Cicely, fighting her feelings.

"It wouldn't be too arduous a job while you're still convalescent," went on Dr Elliott, "and you know such a lot about diet."

Cicely composed herself and managed to smile. "Of course if you want me to be dietician, then I will be."

It was an important job, she told herself firmly. She emphasised this in her mind and tried to suppress the unbearable feelings about not having any children to look after.

"Margaret is a mother herself," she said staunchly, "and separated from her own children. I'm sure that knowing this will help the other mothers."

"What about the medical services generally?" she asked as soon as she had regained her composure.

"Difficult," said Dr Elliott. "We had our first death this morning, and I'm afraid there will be more during the next few days. We have no insulin, and a couple of diabetics are already in a bad way. Look," she pointed out of the window, "there's the coffin in the courtyard."

In the courtyard women were making litttle crosses of grass and laying them on the coffin.

"It's one of the most pathetic sights I've ever seen."

"The grass cross becomes a symbol of our tradition," said Dr Elliott. She crossed herself and bowed momentarily in prayer.

But Cicely felt aggressive. "Grass crosses mean that one

isn't abandoning one's traditions. Survival depends on fighting every inch of the way."

That moment roused in her the overpowering desire to fight which became a cornerstone for survival, as prayer might be for others. Later, when she was taken by the Secret Police, the feeling was even stronger. She learnt that she had to keep up her antagonism in order to survive. It didn't matter whether it did any good or not. It was something inside her that she had to obey.

The nights are the worst, thought Cicely some weeks later, lying on her mattress on the concrete slab of her bed-squatter. So she tried to think about the days. Really, they were not too bad and passed busily. But it always came to the nights. One trouble was the shut-in feeling, though this wore off after a time. Another trouble was nightmares. Cicely seldom suffered in this way herself, but she was distressed to hear the other women screaming in night terrors. They would also pull the chains of their bed-squatters and wake everyone up. Every sound seemed to echo down the iron staircases and reverberate along the corridors, running round the cells until it seemed to create a clanging, screaming hell.

"What are we going to do about it?" asked Patricia Elliott, despairing. "We must stop people behaving like this. It damages everyone."

"It's a question of people learning to limit activity and to live in a community," said Cicely. "Some find it much more difficult than others. If you watch people you see that many go through phases. For a while they're very gallant and help other people. Then for a while they're bloody-minded and a nuisance to everyone. Then again they go into a better phase. Nearly everyone has periods of being irrational. Shhhhh . . . Listen to the argument across the way."

Raised voices floated across the partition.

"The British let us down. If Singapore had capitulated earlier we shouldn't have had to go through all the bombing and destruction."

"I don't agree. If only we'd been more efficient we could have held out for much longer and we shouldn't be in this mess now."

"You often hear people arguing like that," said Dr Elliott.

"It's a way of getting rid of bitterness," said Cicely. "To some the situation is much more damaging than to others, and it's interesting how some seem to take it as a sort of challenge and even enjoy it. Yet others seem to be in constant despair."

"Work helps," said Dr Elliott. "Everyone who is fit should have some. We try to organise it but it's difficult."

"You never know what acute stresses people are going through at certain times," said Cicely, "and if you make allowances for them it helps." This became one of her soothing remarks whenever someone exploded about someone else.

"What do you find most difficult, Cicely?"

She thought for a moment, and then answered, "Having the same people with the same old bloody monotony all the time. It's the monotony of their problems, the monotony of some of their egos, and the impossibility of getting away from it all."

"You conceal your feelings."

But at times she felt intolerant of everyone round her, or sometimes of a particular person until she could stand the sight of her no longer. Then for a while she would take her pudding basin and have meals alone in her cell.

The Japanese sentries and camp officers wandered in and out of the women's quarters at all times, which was much worse for the prisoners at night. The Japanese would come sneaking along the corridor in their rubber shoes. At the door of the women's quarters they would shout, march in, stamp, and stamp out again. Anyone who didn't get up and bow at once was slapped in the face or kicked. One woman had lost a leg in a motor accident, and because she was slow to get up from the floor she was hit hard and often.

"They're so inhuman," said Eleanor Hopkins, one of the women doctors. "How can they behave like this?"

"I think it's a deliberate policy," said Cicely. "They mean to disturb us. I think that we should try to understand it as that."

"I have never imposed my position as the wife of a judge, but I do think someone might give me the lid of the dustbin."

The dignified upper-class voice floated incongruously down the corridor. Cicely was talking to Freddie Bloom, a young and newly married woman with whom she was becoming friendly. They both laughed.

"Mrs Murray Ainsley," said Freddie. "Hasn't she done the dustbin parade yet?"

"It's fascinating," said Cicely speculatively, "how emptying a dustbin can become so important to the wife of a high official who's never had to lift a finger in her life."

The dustbin parade, apart from being the means of garbage disposal, was also an illicit means of communication between the two sides of the prison. Every day the women took their dustbins to the courtyard and the men came to collect them. This involved such deep feeling that it had to be strictly organised. An ex-school mistress, Miss Foss, had been put in charge. She organised it so that a woman could hand over her dustbin to her husband. Everyone who had a bit of lipstick left or a pretty blouse would put it on for the occasion.

"How do you think we shall describe our lives here in prison when we get home to our friends and relatives?" asked Freddie. Her husband was in the military section of Changi, which had no official communication with the civilian prisoners.

Cicely hesitated, and then said, "I suppose the dominant features are discomfort, noise, overcrowding and queuing, bowing to the Japanese and inadequate food."

What she really wanted to talk about was hope, but this she did not dare to do because hope was becoming distorted and even ugly. For one of the big difficulties was the uncertainty of the future and the fact that no one could face it. It seemed that no one ever dared to think that imprisonment could last longer than another three months at the most. Later this confidence seemed pathetic, but she realised that it had been both their salvation and their ruin. They were always thinking about release and repatriation, and only in their gloomiest moments did they indulge in long-distance planning.

She was so conscious of this that she began to discipline herself in an attempt to look ahead, but she could envisage nothing except a sticky end and it was impossible to discuss this with other people. She felt that if the Allies were winning the Japanese would kill the prisoners. If the Japanese were winning they would still kill the prisoners and no one would ask any questions. She could not envisage Allied troops entering as conquering heroes.

One woman refused to go into a certain quadrangle. It gave her the shivers, she said. Cicely never said anything to her or to anybody else, but she always imagined that when the Japanese put them down they would line them up against that particular wall.

For all that there were moments of rare delight, perhaps a new mattress, a valued book or a night in the compound à la belle étoile.

"At least they don't assault us sexually," said Cicely, changing the subject to shift her thoughts.

"They don't find European women attractive," said Freddie. "They don't like our smell."

"Isn't anyone having an affair with a Jap?"

"Yes, but mostly non-Europeans."

"What do they get in return?"

"Food mostly, I think. Particularly food for their children."

"Oh, come and look," called another woman, pointing out of the window. "There's something so funny to watch. A Japanese is trying to ride a horse."

"The ones I've seen aren't exactly expert horsemen," said Cicely, moving to the window.

Outside a Japanese soldier was wobbling dangerously on the back of a good natured cavalry horse. Cicely and Freddie arrived in time to see him fall off. "Hooray," called Freddie, clapping.

"Oh," cried Cicely, "how killingly funny. He's slapping the horse's face just as they slap ours when we don't do what they want. Oh God, they are absurd. At times I feel almost motherly towards the Japanese."

"I'm sorry, Cicely, I'll have to ask you to move out of your cell. I need it for two, maybe even three mothers and babies. I know it's a terrible thing to do to you, but I've nowhere else to put them."

The committee that organised "accommodation" was obviously unhappy to deprive Cicely of her valued privacy, and Cicely hastened to reassure them.

"Oh, I don't mind. I've been marvellously lucky to have the bed-squatter during my convalescence, and now I shall be all right in the corridor. I came here from hospital, where life was much worse. Also, I have things which not everyone has—a mattress, for instance, and a mug and spoon, and a couple of empty tins to carry my food. I even have some money to buy clothes."

Dr Elliott was pleased and said, "We've managed to persuade the Japanese to agree to a shopping expedition tomorrow—aiming at food and clothes. You had better come on it."

Apart from overcrowding, conditions improved slowly. At first all outside supplies were forbidden, even the coconuts that grew just outside the prison walls. The only food was rice and a small stock of tins. But gradually more was supplied, and occasionally lorries and ambulances were allowed to leave the prison. Food and clothes were still obtainable at a price in Singapore.

Occasionally Cicely was allowed to go to the men's side of the camp to arrange with her opposite number about food. He was a cheerful man, and she always felt better after seeing him.

"Have you noticed the noises made by the Japanese when they're angry?" he asked one day. He used the same tone of voice as in discussing rice rations so as not to arouse the suspicion of the Japanese guard in the corner.

"Yes, I have," said Cicely. "The noise defies all description. Until you've heard it you don't believe that a human being could make it."

"I knew it reminded me of something," he said, "and now I realise what it is. I've been allowed out recently to do some gardening. The other day I was weeding my plot when I heard close behind me the sound of an angry Japanese. As you know, they always get mad with anger if one doesn't leap to one's feet instantly and bow. So I did. But when I had finished all the bowing and scraping and actually looked up I found it wasn't a Japanese at all. It was a dog being sick."

Cicely laughed. "That's exactly what it sounds like," she said.

One afternoon she sat on her mattress in the few feet of corridor that was now her home. Jeanette, a young friend who was a keen gardener, passed down the corridor, stopped and said, "It wouldn't be bad here if it weren't for the Japs."

This sort of joke was made too often to be funny. Cicely went straight to the point.

"What's the matter?"

"The Japanese don't like us growing vegetables and flowers. We've got to pull them all up." She stamped her foot.

"Shame," said Cicely soothingly. "Just when urine and sludge were beginning to give such good results. I must say, internment is wonderful for resourcefulness. Look at this."

She smiled and held out her glasses. "New frames," she said proudly.

Jeanette was incredulous. "How on earth . . .?"

"Sent over from the men's side, a special present from a very inventive craftsman," said Cicely. "They're made out of an old toothbrush handle. They have also sent us some marvellous 'plaster' bandages made out of latex. It means that we can actually *do* something for our patients—the ones that need plaster, that is."

The Medical Committee, one of the many committees formed by the prisoners, had already organised a "hospital" with a sick bay for "in-patients" and a clinic for "out-patients".

The sick bay was soon filled with old people, many of whom died, and the doctors could do little to help. The out-patient department was busy, not only with day to day problems of established internees but also with vetting new arrivals.

"I sometimes wondered about that," said Jeannette. "What can you actually do for your patients? Have you any drugs, for instance?"

"We have hardly anything," said Cicely. She had already learnt how easy it was to keep on just seeing patients and giving advice without attempting to evaluate what was happening.

"I suppose we mostly give uplift and a hot water bottle. If, of course, we can get any hot water. I imagine that my most important medical job at the moment is to advise on how we use our food supply."

"That reminds me," said Jeannette. "I've heard some good news. The Japanese have given permission for the men to do all the cooking."

"Thank God," said Cicely. The Committee had worked hard for this. Not only did the men have the kitchens on their side of the prison, but they also went out with the lorries and were in a better position to find food.

"I must go," she said. "It's time for my weighing session." Wearing her new glasses she walked down the corridor with a lighter step than for some time.

She held a weighing session in the out-patients every afternoon, and each woman came once a month. She knew that the women enjoyed this. It gave them a chance to talk, and Cicely could study their health and their reactions. She tried to tell herself that the whole experience was a privilege. Here she was, a trained observer under extraordinary conditions, with superb opportunites to study how she and other people felt and behaved. It made her feel that she must not only accept the inevitability but even welcome it.

"I don't seem to have lost any weight this month." said the woman standing on the scales. "It must be the 'cow bodies' we had last week."

They both laughed. Their rare issues of meat were always

sent to them from English-speaking Japanese officials under the title "cow bodies".

"Maybe," said Cicely. "I think your body is also getting used to the rice diet. Young people adapt better than older people." Cicely had been keeping careful records of the women's weights, and was interested to watch how they went down. "All the Europeans lost weight at first," she explained. "The older people more rapidly than the younger. But after a while nearly everyone begins to stabilise, and even when food supplies diminish still further people stop losing weight and may even improve. Eurasians and non-Europeans seem to recover more quickly than the Europeans, probably because they are used to a rice diet."

The woman sighed. "My children don't remember what bread is like."

"But the children in this camp are vigorous and cheerful," said Cicely, encouraging her.

"Not everyone is well. My sister is very sick."

Cicely knew that the sister was dying. "People react so differently," she said gently.

Some couldn't take it at all and died. Others swelled up or became so dizzy that they had to stay in bed. Nearly everyone had beri-beri or anaemia or both. But on the whole Cicely was surprised how tough people were, and how they managed to go through periods of near-starvation without suffering more.

The next woman had lost weight and was upset and demanding.

"I've heard you have some tonic medicine, Doctor. Don't you think I ought to have some?"

"I have no tonics, and only a few drugs for emergencies."

"That's not what I heard," said the woman, raising her voice.

"I'm sorry. I can't help what you heard."

"But I think I ought to have some all the same."

"I'm sorry," said Cicely again. "I'm afraid I don't agree."

"But my periods have stopped, Doctor. I'm in a terrible state of health."

"Everyone's periods have stopped," said Cicely.

It was one of the odd things about the camp life. Nearly all the women stopped menstruating immediately on arrival in camp, long before the change of diet could have had any effect. Cicely realised that this must be due to psychological shock. After the war she discovered that the same thing had happened in concentration camps in other parts of the world.

"Then I can't have any medicine?" The woman was angry now.

Cicely sighed. Some people were very demanding. They felt that they couldn't miss anything that was going.

"No, I'm afraid you can't."

She got rid of her with difficulty, and was thankful that the clinic was at an end.

On her way back through the corridor she saw a queue forming, and without thinking she joined it. Queuing had become a habit, for everything and for every meal. But nothing happened. She turned to her next-door neighbour and said, "What are we queuing for? Coconuts?" "No," replied the other woman. "This is the queue for confession."

"Come," said a laughing woman sitting at a table near by. She was staring at a small round object.

"Good Heavens," Cicely said. "That looks like a cake."

The woman beamed. "It is a cake."

"However . . . ? Whatever . . . ?" Cicely scarcely knew how to ask.

The woman laughed. "I found a bit of rice that someone had thrown into the rubbish bin, so I scraped it out and dried it and pounded it into flour, and I found an egg that someone had dropped on the floor, so I scraped that up, and I happened to have a bit of sugar and this is the result."

The cake was only about four inches across, but the woman cut a small piece for Cicely to taste.

"It's delicious," Cicely said, almost truthfully.

She was becoming obsessed with thoughts of food, and suffered more from this than from the physical discomfort of feeling hungry or even of finding herself becoming weaker and weaker and not knowing how long she would be able to carry on. She knew that everyone else had the same feeling. They couldn't read, talk or think of anything without the idea of food coming to mind. And it had to be nice food too. Hence the rice that the woman had found in the dustbin. She came to understand how starving people can throw away food because it smells bad or even because it isn't what they want to eat at that moment. This was particularly true of the children, who often became resentful and refused to look at unaccustomed food.

One evening, while resting on her concrete slab, she heard the sing-song Spanish voice of Mrs Palomar.

"And this is how you make *paella* . . ."

It was the beginning of a craze for writing out recipes. Everyone exchanged them and made notes for delicious cookery. Complicated and sophisticated recipes were particularly in demand, and of these the Spanish and Dutch women seemed to have the greatest store.

Many women wanted to keep diaries too, though some admitted that it was only to write about food. But paper was a problem. Every scrap was needed for official and medical records and for the children's schooling.

The days passed busily. There were committees for nearly everything and these took up much time, as did education for the children, concerts in the quadrangles and lectures on whatever anyone could be found to talk about. A Russian prima donna, married to a British judge, organised singing classes. Many people spent much of the day playing bridge or mah jong. Some people made packs of cards from the backs of matchboxes, but eventually matches were even scarcer than cards. There were a few books, and these were very much at a premium.

"Have you heard? The Archdeacon's wife died this morning."

"But she's been here such a short while."

"There's only one coffin left."

"Can't we get any more?"

"No one's going to use our precious wood to make coffins."

"It seems dreadful. So many people die."

"They'll take the coffin to the burial and then bring it back again."

"We're all becoming brutalised. It's one of the worst things. None of us will be fit for civilised society again."

"What are they doing about the Archdeacon?" asked Cicely, breaking into the conversation. She felt deeply anxious about him.

"They're letting him come over from the men's side to officiate."

"What a way for a marriage to end," said someone, sitting with head bowed in the corner.

The Archdeacon arrived and his face was gaunt and strained. He wore his surplice and a bright blue stole.

"I will go alone," he said, walking towards the lorry that carried his wife's body. Cicely watched him climb up laboriously and drive away. It was one of the few occasions during all those years in prison when she cried.

The Archdeacon himself died three weeks later. He had only been in prison for a few months, and Cicely knew that she would never forget the circumstances of his arrival or the powerful feelings it raised in her.

A few weeks earlier a fellow prisoner had said, "Are you religious, Cicely?"

"Not really, though I think it's a good prop. I actually like going to church. It seems a way of recharging the batteries. But I can't really claim to be religious."

All the same, since she had been in prison she had had deep feelings about religion and a yearning for some kind of ritual.

"We're going to be allowed to have a service."

"Marvellous." She was delighted. Most of the Anglican clergy were still free. She had been much to the fore in trying to persuade the Japanese to allow one of them to come to the prison to hold a service.

"Who's coming?" she asked.

"Archdeacon Graham White. But he's been told he mustn't preach a sermon."

"Well, he can read from the liturgy instead and we'll all enjoy that," said Cicely.

When she saw the Archdeacon arrive for the service she had a feeling in her throat that was difficult to reconcile with her lack of religious beliefs. The women filed into the largest room in the prison and sat on the bare concrete wherever they could find a space, mostly on the floor. There was an echoing silence, and a sense of awe filled the room as the Archdeacon arrived. Tall and dignified, he picked his way slowly among them.

"Let us pray."

His voice rang out, and its elegant articulation could have come from another world.

When it came to the part of the service where the lesson is usually read the Archdeacon seemed to straighten himself to an immense height before speaking in a steady, deliberate voice. Cicely waited, conscious of an overwhelming feeling of suspense through the whole gathering.

"I will now read Psalm 79. Oh God, the heathen are come into thine inheritance; thy holy temple have they defiled; they have laid Jerusalem on heaps. The dead bodies of thy servants have they given to be meat unto the fowls of the heaven, the flesh of thy saints unto the beasts of the land. Their blood have they shed like water round about Jerusalem; and there was none to bury them. We are become a reproach to our neighbours, a scorn and derision to them that are round about us. Let the sighing of the prisoner come before thee; according to the greatness of thy power preserve thou those that are appointed to die."

Cicely felt it was lucky that the Japanese guard did not understand English.

Shortly after this, without realising it, she glimpsed her own future.

She fell ill again and had to go back to the Myako Hospital, which was now Japanese. There she saw her old friend Maud Pereira, who, being Sinhalese, had not been interned and was looking after the children in the wards. When she was convalescent Cicely visited these wards. She thought that by now she was numb to horror, yet the sight of her former patients distressed her more than she had anticipated. The Japanese were not providing food for the children, or enough staff. Many of them were rapidly deteriorating.

She turned away and gazed down the ward to where a nurse was arranging bottles in rows with mechanical movements without raising her head. She looked old and defeated, yet somehow familiar.

"She reminds me of Nurse Benjamin," said Cicely.

"It is Nurse Benjamin," said Mrs Pereira.

"Whatever has happened to her?" asked Cicely, horrified. "She looks twenty years older."

"She has been in serious trouble with the Japanese," said Mrs Pereira quietly. "They sent her to what they call the Kempaitai, the military police or Gestapo. I don't know what happened to her there. She won't talk about it."

Quietly Cicely moved down the ward and confronted her former nurse. Nurse Benjamin looked up, gave a half smile of recognition, then turned away sobbing.

"Doctor, Doctor, it was terrible. Terrible."

Later Cicely discovered what it was really like because she was sent there herself.

CHAPTER X

When Cicely had been in prison for some months a rumour spread.

"Asahi is letting the Eurasians out on parole and even trying to persuade them to go."

Asahi was the Japanese in control of all the enemy aliens in Singapore, including the camp. When the rumour turned out to be true Cicely felt that it confirmed something she had come to believe. Basically Asahi was a decent man.

He came in person one day, small, neat and polite. He spoke to the Eurasians and tried to persuade them to take parole. But after he had gone many expressed uncertainty and fear.

"If we go, who knows what they may do? We may land in trouble in Singapore. At least we're protected here."

"But if we go out we can help our own people far more than we can here."

"I believe Asahi is really trying to help," said Cicely, encouragingly. "He is genuinely concerned about the overcrowding here."

Many of the Eurasians went. Soon afterwards they heard that Asahi wanted six men to work in his office in Singapore. He announced, "This will not compromise you. Mine is the office for enemy aliens. I need secretarial help." It was clear to Cicely that he did not really need the men. Again this seemed to be a genuine attempt to help the prisoners.

Next day she heard that Asahi now wanted two doctors, a man and a woman, to go out and live in Singapore, work in his office, and write reports for him on the diet of Europeans in Singapore before the war and the diets of everybody since.

"You're the obvious person, Cicely."

"Oh no," she said diffidently. "I'm sure there are others who would be better than me."

But there obviously weren't, and she was selected unanimously.

On a steamy Sunday morning she and Doctor Eric Byron, who had been selected by the men, were driven out of prison in a lorry together with the men chosen to be clerks. They were taken to Singapore, where they were bundled into Fullerton Building, the Government Administrative Office. To Cicely's surprise they were marched straight into what had been the office of the Medical Officer.

"What a change," she muttered under her breath to Doctor Byron.

She had known the office before the Japanese invasion. In those days it had been filled with stacks of files and busy people running in and out. What she now saw made her want to giggle.

All round the walls were tables, and at each sat a Japanese soldier staring straight ahead with a sheet of clean pink blotting paper in front of him and nothing else. A long screaming conversation took place between the guard and the blotting paper soldiers. Then the seven men prisoners and Cicely were marched into Asahi's office, where they lined up in front of him and bowed. He made no response.

For several minutes he did not lift his head. They had learnt long ago that a Japanese method to keep people in subjection was to ignore them.

Eventually he looked up and they bowed again. A faint smile seemed to cross his face as he started to speak.

"When the Japanese took Singapore and renamed it *Shyonan*,* the military decided that you should all disappear." He flapped his right hand at them all and continued. "But my Emperor decided that you should not disappear and he gave me the work of looking after you. For me this is not very constructive work. But it is what my Emperor has told me to do and I will do it as best I can."

* Rising Sun.

The Europeans bowed again and waited for what was to come.

"I have lived in England for some time," he said, "and I know the English. I have ordered you to come here and work in my office. For you this is not compromising. You will be working to help your own people." And again he said, "I have lived in England. I have great deal respect of English gentleman and lady." At this point they all bowed. "And while you are working for me on parole in Singapore I have confidence that you will obey obligations of parole and do nothing that would disgrace you or me, English gentlemen and lady."

"I think that's a fair statement of the position," said Cicely to Dr Byron when they were once more in the lorry. "Have you any idea where we shall live?"

"In the Post Office, I should think," said Byron. "I gather that all the Europeans who are still at large live there. The only exceptions are the Bishop and two other padres, who have a house to themselves."

In the Post Office Cicely was given a small flat, with two beds and bare essentials. The men lived in big wards elsewhere in the building. At Cicely's door there was always a burly Sikh guard. She was told that she could have no visitors, and was given 50 Malayan dollars with which to feed herself for a month.

It was dangerous, she knew, to come out of prison on parole. In the town it was easy to get into trouble, and there were many temptations. Not least of these was the desire to find out what was really going on. If someone had forecast Cicely's future she would not have been surprised to hear that her lips would be sewn up with wire as a punishment for listening to the foreign radio, or that pencils would be stuck into her head, the punishment for those caught listening to the B.B.C. or repeating the news. When she crossed Fullerton Bridge and saw the long metal spikes displaying the heads of those caught resisting the Japanese, she knew that her own head might soon join them.

But if someone had predicted that she would, of her own accord, lunch at the house of a Japanese professor, drive with him in public and sit with him drinking orange squash in the Botanical Gardens, she would not have believed it. She had already learnt that collaboration and resistance are often not simple matters of black and white, but she had not yet experienced the depth of duplicity which may apply to each, or the difficulties that anyone outside an immediate situation may have in deciphering its significance.

She knew that living out of prison was likely to be a tightrope existence. At a small false move she could lose her head or worse. Yet even such minimum friendliness as might be necessary to avoid arrest could be misconstrued by her fellow Europeans and cause trouble later. On top of all this the Japanese, with their different background and culture, were liable to react in unexpected ways.

Later, reflecting in less happy circumstances on the whole sequence of events, she realised that it would probably not have been possible to return from parole unscathed. But she never regretted her decision to go out into Singapore, for it had given her new opportunities to help her fellow-prisoners.

She was allowed no visitors, but she received invitations, first from her friends the Zehnders and then from the Bishop himself. Yet she did not go anywhere of her own accord. She would go first to Asahi and ask permission. "People have invited me. I tell you first so that you know that I am open." And Asahi would say, "You can go." And, lighthearted then, she went.

She discovered her mistake too late. Every visit she made to her old friends was marked up against her.

One day, as every day, she sat writing her report at her table in Asahi's office. Beside her sat Dr Eric Byron writing his. They were the only Europeans in the office; the others had been put elsewhere in the building. All round the wall sat Japanese men in uniform, staring, unmoving, and not apparently engaged in any form of activity. The only sound came from Eric Byron's pen, which squeaked.

Cicely fingered the enormous label on her blouse, which displayed her photograph and a statement that she was an enemy alien and very wicked. They were all forced to wear these labels as part of the Japanese campaign to humiliate the Europeans in front of the people of Singapore.

She was trying to write her report slowly, to spin out this period of semi-freedom. It is not easy to slow up work that comes easily to an active, interested mind, and she had to invent ploys and mental tricks to prolong it, such as recopying what was already neatly written, polishing and repolishing the grammar and syntax.

Eric Byron caught her eye with an expression that suggested lunch. Cicely smiled. This was the best moment of the day. Although they were closely guarded they were allowed out for an hour to buy food in the market or to eat in one of the little Indian or Chinese restaurants.

They stood up and bowed to the Japanese guards, making a point, as part of their subtle methods of resistance, not to bow in unison. They received no response but, feeling that they could now avoid arousing the hostility of their captors, walked out into the hot street.

Byron, like the other men, wore only a G-string and had no other clothes. He was lean and brown like a Malay, and this was also part of the Japanese policy of humiliation. During the great march of the families from Singapore out to Changi the Japanese had been hoping that the Chinese would enjoy the Europeans' humiliation and add to it. But in fact people stood in the streets with tears running down their faces and ran out of their houses with glasses of water, and some went down on their knees and prayed that they might go safely.

They stopped at a banana stall and Cicely chose a small bunch, all that she felt she could afford. The Chinese market man looked carefully left and right, pushed them into her hands and whispered, "No pay. No pay". The expression of compassion on his face made Cicely feel warm and full of hope.

"Look at that," said Dr Byron, pointing. Along the road sped an open truck, packed with thin brown men, some in khaki shorts and some only in G-strings. Cicely looked closely and saw that they were British prisoners, probably being transported for coolie work.

A small Chinese boy ran out of a near-by building with one hand behind his back. He too looked first one way and then the other. Having made sure that no Japanese were looking he hurled a small object, possibly a tin of sardines, into the lorry. One of the prisoners caught it with a smile and waved at the boy as the lorry swept on.

Cicely looked up and found another European beside her. She knew that he was a policeman, but she did not know his name or why he was out on parole.

"This is dangerous," he said. "You don't know what you're getting involved in. You had much better go back to prison."

"No," said Eric Byron, with the anger of fear not confronted.

Cicely wanted to change the subject and said, "Quick, it's going to rain."

"Rickshaw?" called a rickshaw puller in the street, pointing at the rapidly darkening sky.

Cicely wanted to get away so badly that she scarcely noticed when the rickshaw puller showed the characteristic Chinese attitude towards Europeans and refused to take any payment.

"For God's sake," said Cicely. "This is most dangerous."

Her friend, Edith Zehnder, carefully rolled up the slip of paper on which was written B.B.C. News and stuffed it back in the little hole by her electric light.

"You must be mad," said Cicely. "If anybody gives it to you, read it. Then for heaven's sake tear it up."

But Edith laughed. She told Cicely that she was going to organise a rebellion and that she had five hundred Union Jacks under her floor. Her friends among the Chinese shopkeepers and other people were going to help her.

Cicely felt too frightened to go to the Zehnders' again.

Not long after she heard that the Japanese had searched their house. But luckily Edith had been warned in time and had burnt the Union Jacks under leaves in her garden.

One day Cicely plucked up courage and went to Asahi and

said, "It is not correct for a woman to live alone like this. I also need someone to do my typing if I am going to write this report. I suggest that you bring Mrs de Moubray out of prison to help me. She can type and we can live together and it will be far more correct."

To her surprise he agreed, and after a week Katherine came. They lived together in the Post Office flat and Cicely found this much more fun.

"What are we going to do when this is finished?" asked Katherine one day, looking up from her typewriter.

Cicely had worked on her report in a leisurely manner but even so, after six weeks, it was nearly finished.

"I don't know," she answered. "Asahi seems to be willing for us to go on pottering about his office without a specific job for as long as we want. But I don't like the prospect."

She knew that the longer she stayed out on parole the more likely she was to get into serious trouble with the Japanese. There was already a rumour that the cultural authorities of the Japanese were going to ask them to do some other work.

"What about the library?" asked Katherine.

"I've been wondering about that."

She felt that there were two aims that she might achieve in the library. One was somehow to arrange for books to be sent to Changi prison, where the shortage of books was impeding the children's education and causing suffering to the more educated prisoners. The other aim was purely private, though she felt that it was also needed by the prison community. She had lost all her medical notes, and was anxious to do some medical reading. Many problems had arisen in camp, and she wanted to read up a number of subjects.

"Have you found out what has happened to the books?" asked Katherine. All the libraries, private and public, had been emptied by the Japanese.

"They haven't been destroyed yet," said Cicely. "Apparently they're all in the Raffles Museum and two Englishmen are working there, trying to rescue them."

"Can we go there?"

"I gather that the books aren't available to anyone except through the personal permission of Professor Tanakadate. He's a Japanese who has been appointed as Head of the Raffles Museum and is sort of Head of Culture in Singapore."

She tried to get in touch with him. The answer was an invitation to lunch. It soon became clear that Professor Tanakadate wanted to be friendly. Cicely and Katherine refused. He asked them to lunch again and again. They lost count of the number of times. Each time they refused. Then one day Asahi told them that Tanakadate wanted them to go and work at the Raffles Museum. They were worried, and knew that if they accepted it might lead to trouble. On the other hand the camp needed books urgently, and this was a possible means of getting them. They went to the Bishop and asked what they should do about it. He said, "My principle is to be friendly with everyone in the world, as friendly as you possibly can. I don't think there is any harm in being friendly. It doesn't matter what anybody says."

So, after a good deal of heart-searching, they decided to accept the job and go and work at the Raffles Museum.

"Do you think they are collaborators?" asked Katherine, referring to the two Europeans who were already working in the Raffles Museum.

"No," said Cicely firmly, "though I can see that it must look like that to many people. They may seem to be co-operating with the enemy, but I think you could regard it as an opportunity to carry on useful work and keep up the spirits of people outside. One of the things we're learning the hard way is that relationships with an enemy conqueror are not simple. It's impossible to say what is collaboration and what is reasonable lack of hostility, and what is justified and what is not. And people so seldom agree. Some play difficult and complicated double games, and I shall never blame anyone for collaborating because I know that some of the people who I have felt were collaborating were, in fact, performing dangerous and subtle roles in this whole beastly business of war. And it's all complicated by the pathetic anxiety of the Japanese to be friendly. It's difficult for a conqueror to be dignified."

As soon as they had started work at the Raffles Museum, Tanakadate renewed his invitation to lunch. They both thought him a sly old man and didn't like him. But Cicely realised that he could do a lot for the prisoners in Changi and that he was prepared to do so.

She consulted the Bishop again and he said, "Go." With qualms she and Katherine eventually accepted the invitation, and this was how they came to drive with him in the Botanical Gardens and drink orange pop at a kiosk. His aim was obviously to advertise the fact that Europeans were friendly with him. They heard that the week before he had been called upon to show three Japanese generals round the Gardens, and they had also demanded to sit in the open and drink orange pop. "It might have had a good effect on the Malayan campaign," he said, "if it had been possible for three British generals to drink orange pop in the Botanical Gardens."

While they sat there fraternising they started to work on him. Cicely said, "Our children are growing up in prison. They don't even know that there are roots to trees. They see only concrete walls around them. The men can go out on rice fatigues or cutting wood. But the women never go outside the walls and neither do the children." They asked, couldn't they occasionally go outside, couldn't they sometimes have meetings with the men? Since February wives and husbands had not been able to see each other. Would it be possible to arrange meetings?

His reply was, "Japanese soldiers left home as long as two years ago. They do not even write letters. If one child is starving you do not show him another child eating a nice juicy apple."

"Well," Katherine told him, "that is for them to arrange, but it is hard that people do not see each other when it could be arranged. And there is another thing too. The prisoners would like to have letters because they have had none from home. And, furthermore, your soldiers are collecting all these books in the Museum, sometimes as many as 200 copies of David Copperfield or Shakespeare. The Japanese don't need these and they are no use to anyone in the Museum." She asked, couldn't they sort out the books and send them both to the military and to the civilian internees so that they would have something to read? This would not disturb the Japanese at all.

All the requests that Cicely and Katherine made that day were granted within two months. But they paid a heavy price. When they got back to camp it was held against them that they had fraternised with the Japanese. Later, when Cicely was taken by the Kempaitai, it was held against her that she had seen people and had had contacts in Singapore.

But as a result of her "fraternisation" there was a library of 3,000 books in Changi prison for the internees, and more for the prisoners-of-war. She was convinced that this made an enormous difference, not only to people's lives but also to their survival.

As Christmas approached Cicely and Katherine felt growing enjoyment and fear. They were surprised and pleased to get permission to have parties with the men. There was also a Nativity play in the church, and they sang in the choir. It was the only time that Cicely saw the three wise men played by men of different races, Chinese, Indian and Malay.

But in the background all the time was the noise floating through the windows of the Raffles Museum. The Museum was only about two hundred yards from the Y.M.C.A., now the headquarters of the Kempaitai, the Japanese Gestapo. There was no doubt about how the Kempaitai treated its victims.

In the middle of January, suddenly, without warning, they were sent back into Changi prison.

Another woman doctor, Eleanor Hopkins, was now head of the women's camp.

"Things have settled in Changi quite a lot," she said. "We have organised a school on the women's side and a university on the men's."

"There must be many highly educated men over there," said Cicely.

"Indeed, yes, and they are running a variety of courses with infinite ingenuity, even in practical science. Their 'apparatus' for the laboratory includes old electric light bulbs cut off near the brass cap, which make excellent boiling flasks. They've got quicklime by burning coral which they picked up on the beach, and I'm told that laxative tablets contain enough phenolphthalein to use as chemical indicators."

"Can we women benefit from all this?"

"Oh yes. Men come over several times a week to lecture here in the women's camp."

"It's marvellous to find this rise in intellectual standards," said Cicely, genuinely pleased.

"And I've got some good news for you, Cicely. At least, I hope you will take it as such. There is a special request from the men that as soon as you are back in camp we arrange for you to go over and lecture to them. They want a series on child health, and I gather you'll have an audience of at least forty doctors."

She was delighted. It didn't occur to her either that she would be the only woman who lectured in the men's camp or that this might in any way be held against her. Later she discovered that the Kempaitai had other views.

Soon after Cicely's return to prison the Japanese asked Dr Eleanor Hopkins to resign. Apparently her manner annoyed them in some way. So there was an election and Cicely got in by a few votes. In some ways she was frightened of doing the job, but she also saw that it would be interesting. It meant going to all the men's committee meetings and fencing a good deal with the Japanese. This was quite fun in spite of the unpleasantness of being yelled at and having revolvers waved at her. It also meant dealing with people, often at their worst, in difficult and intimate situations, and this she found hardest of all, but also the most interesting. Some people, she found, had extraordinary concepts about their duties, responsibilities and rights, and this could make a great deal of difference to how they reacted in prison and what they expected from the head of the camp. It became a private game to guess what her fellow prisoners were like in ordinary life. She suspected that most people in prison behaved much as they did outside. But this was certainly not always so. For instance, some of the idle wives of officials, who had done nothing but sit around all their lives, gave willing hands to menial tasks. Often they positively enjoyed it, and seemed to find a new fulfilment. By contrast, some people seemed to be reliable and then turned out not to be so.

In difficult times she tried to increase her tolerance by assessing her personal reaction to prison life. She told herself how lucky she was, and that it was easier for her than for many others. She was middle-aged and knew how much worse it would have been to be eighteen or nineteen, or a young wife separated from her husband and perhaps eventually hearing that he had died two years before. There were also mothers who were always afraid that their children would starve to death or be executed out of hand. Many had ghastly anxieties that she was spared. There was no one in the camp with whom she was emotionally involved, and she had nothing special to lose by being there, having no great fondness for golf, alcohol or promotion. Moreover, she had a more varied internment than most people, not only because of her period on parole, but also because she was working at an interesting job that she was trained to do.

"The whole experience is a privilege," she told herself firmly.

In this way, for a brief period, life wasn't bad.

One morning she had finished her administrative duties as head of the women's camp and was on her way to the clinic, where she still liked to do as much doctoring as possible. In the corridor she met an acquaintance, who said: "Doctor Williams, I was just coming to find you. There's an urgent summons. The committee must all go to Asahi's office at once."

She hurried upstairs, and found not only the women's committee but also the men's. She took this to be an ominous sign. It must mean that Asahi had an important announcement to make, and she felt sure that it could not be to their advantage. Things had been so much better lately that any change was likely to be for the worse.

They lined up silently in front of Asahi and bowed. As usual he made no acknowledgement, and remained for several minutes with his head down. Then he looked up, and Cicely was struck by the sadness on his face.

"I have a serious announcement to make," he said. "I am leaving. I warn you to be careful in your behaviour, because I think you will find that things will change." He wished them well, Cicely made a brief, polite reply, and they filed out silently, exchanging glances of anxiety and fear.

Later that morning Cicely had to take some papers to Asahi's office. On the way upstairs she met him coming down. She flattened herself against the wall, prepared to bow as he passed. But to her surprise he stopped beside her.

He looked carefully up the stairs, then down, and when he was sure that no one was about he took her by the hand and began to cry.

"I pray God," he said, "to take me home safely to my country and you safely to yours. I think you will find that my successor is very different."

It occurred to Cicely that he was being sacked for being too gentle with the prisoners. She felt deeply moved. Only later did she realise the possible implications for their future.

She knew that things would get worse and tried to shut out the thought by working even harder, both as a doctor and as head of the women's camp. It kept her busy all day, especially as she was now slowing up from lack of food.

"Can I play football please, Doctor Williams?"

She looked down at a small eager face and rejoiced that the children, though small and underfed, still had the energy to play football. The little boys lived with their mothers on the women's side, but were allowed over to the men's side once or twice a week to play football.

"I don't know yet, Jimmy. Your knee isn't getting better as quickly as I would like."

"Oh please, Doctor Williams," he pleaded.

Jimmy had twisted his knee the previous week, and Cicely knew how long injuries took to heal under starvation conditions.

"Tell you what," she said. "I'll write a note to a friend of mine over on the men's side, Professor Monro. You go and find him when you get there. He's an expert on knees. If he says you can play, you can. O.K.?"

"O.K.," grinned the child. "I'll find him. I promise."

Cicely wrote on a scrap of paper.

Dear Jack, Please will you see this child because he wants to play football at 2 o'clock. Please examine his knee and don't let him play if he isn't fit.

She wondered whether to add a personal note but decided that it would be too dangerous. To make it look more official she signed it "*Cicely D. Williams, M.D.*"

She reassured herself that the Japanese wouldn't take exception to that, though she knew they could take exception to anything.

"There's been a sinister atmosphere ever since Asahi left," said Katherine, voicing what they all felt.

The camp was now in the charge of a new man, Tominaga. Cicely thought that he looked like a flatulent bullfrog and was out to be as brutal and nasty as he could be. From the day he arrived minor irritations increased.

"Today the funeral ambulance was ready to go to the cemetery and the guards sat smoking for half-an-hour, so it had to wait in the sun for no reason at all."

"They gave us permission to hold a meeting but at the last minute it was cancelled by a sentry."

"How do you get on, Cicely, as head of the camp?"

"It's difficult. Last night I was got out of bed and had to hurry to the office, where they shouted at me because someone hadn't bowed deeply enough to a sentry."

"This bowing business is always causing trouble."

"Yes," said Cicely. "I wish people wouldn't make it the focal point of their resistance. Personally I don't think it's worth worrying about, and I don't care whether I bow to the Japanese front, back or side. But some people never seem to get used to it, and nothing upsets the Japs more quickly."

"Mark my words, there's going to be trouble over the electricity," said a woman prisoner a few days later.

"What makes you think that?"

"I took some shoes for repair in the men's quarters and the cobbler told me. He had it from a man who speaks Japanese and heard them talking about it."

"I suppose we must be using rather a lot of current."

All over the prison now was hidden electrical apparatus, looted from various sources. Cicely had an efficient automatic kettle that Jack Monro had found for her, and other women had irons, frying pans and toasters.

"It's all got to be handed in."

When the expected order came Cicely went to the office and managed to persuade the Japanese officer on duty to allow them to keep a few essentials—one kettle for babies' feeds, one cigarette lighter because there were no matches, one boiling ring for instruments in the sick bay.

He gave her verbal permission but she wondered how much this meant, as he had refused to sign the modest list.

Tominaga spoke fluent English. He said that he was a graduate in psychology of the University of California. But he made the prisoners speak Malay or find an interpreter.

They now began to get the feeling that the Japanese were doing their best to catch them out. There were vindictive punishments. Men were kicked and beaten. Some were locked up without food or water for forty-eight hours. Sometimes a sentry would come into the camp and hit everybody he met.

It wasn't long before Cicely was in serious personal trouble.

One day she was told to go to the office in a hurry. Behind the desk was Kobiashi, one of the nastiest of the Japanese. Behind him were his guards. In front of him was the electrical apparatus which Cicely had been guarding for essential purposes.

Kobiashi screamed at her, tore off her armband and waved a revolver in front of her. "How dare you leave this lying about," he yelled. "You are degraded, and deprived of your appointment."

She knew it was useless to explain that she had kept it with

Japanese permission, or that she hated being head of the camp and didn't mind being demoted. It was useless to say anything at all. She bowed politely, but even this enraged them. She knew then that she would have to go through with whatever they imposed upon her. She felt almost relieved when Kobiashi ordered her to stand in the guard room for twenty-four hours.

The guards on duty at the time were mostly Sikhs, not Japanese. They were rough, but few were hostile, and many retained some consideration for their European prisoners. Some even held that their present job was to care for the Europeans in their charge until times improved.

For several hours Cicely stood vaguely to attention and facing the wall, wondering whether she could do it for twenty-four hours and what would happen about going to the lavatory.

Suddenly a Sikh guard told her to sit down and gave her a cigarette. It turned out that Kobiashi had left the jail and a nicer Japanese was now on duty. Members of the committee had been working on him, and eventually he gave permission for a camp bed, and Cicely spent the rest of her twenty-four hours in moderate comfort.

This incident was typical of the uncertainty and the uneven atmosphere that slowly worsened as though preparing for disaster. Sometimes the Japanese would pounce on some activity hitherto regarded as innocent. Sometimes there was a sudden roll-call, which meant standing for several hours in one of the quadrangles in the blazing sun while Japanese soldiers searched the cells.

"You never know where the hell you are with them," said Mrs Nixon, who was made head of the camp when Cicely was sacked. But her voice struck a deeper, unhappier note. Everyone seemed to feel that something terrible would soon happen, and there was a rumour that it would be on the 10 October.

And in fact the reign of terror began on 10 October 1943, the tenth day of the tenth month of the year. The Double Tenth is a big Chinese feast day, and it was the day chosen by Japan to begin a great swoop on "spies".

A number of Japanese ships had recently been sunk in

Singapore Harbour by Australian soldiers. Dressed as Malay fishermen, they had attached limpet bombs to the hulls. The Japanese suspected that the attack had been organised by prisoners in Changi. They had also been told by informers inside the camp that there were receiving sets in the camp, which was true, and a transmitter, which was not true.

The prisoners went through the same procedure as during previous roll-calls, sitting in the sun all day. It was three o'clock in the afternoon before the roll was actually taken, and some hours later before they were allowed to dismiss. Japanese soldiers came in lorries with guns and bayonets at the ready and examined the cells, the carpenter's and printer's shops and the other big rooms on both sides of the camp.

"They seem determined to accuse us of subversive activities and punish us severely," remarked Freddie Bloom.

"I think we're in for a bad time," said Cicely. "I heard that six or seven radio receivers have been found on the men's side, and more than fifty men prisoners have been arrested and taken into the Kempaitai."

That evening all meetings were stopped and they were told that henceforth groups of more than three or four people were forbidden, including even school for the children.

"Katherine de Moubray has been arrested and taken away by the Kempaitai."

The rumour spread round the camp so fast that it almost echoed in the corridors. Everywhere Cicely noticed white, tense faces.

But an hour later, before they had even recovered, Katherine was back, shaken, bewildered but unhurt. She had been questioned and that was all.

Cicely and Freddie were sitting with her in the corridor trying to comfort and support her when three Japanese soldiers in the uniform of the Secret Police burst through the doors at the end and advanced on them.

"Oh God, what now?" murmured Katherine, at the end of her tether.

The soldiers seized Freddie and marched her down the corridor. Desperate and helpless, Katherine and Cicely ran along beside her until they were pushed and kicked. Katherine cried openly. Cicely just had time to thrust into Freddie's hand a sort of bun of rice and flour which was her ration. It seemed to be an instinct to give something that might help.

"Oh God," said Katherine, slumping into the corner. "What does it all mean?"

"I think I understand now," said Cicely. "I think they arrested you in mistake for Freddie. They probably suspect her because she used to work with the British Information Agency."

The more she thought about this the more certain she felt. But she had hardly worked it out when Eleanor Hopkins came down the corridor and said in a worried voice, "I gather that someone on the men's side was also arrested, questioned and returned. Just like Katherine. He's a doctor. I wonder what it all means?"

"What was his name?" asked Cicely.

"Nearly the same as yours, Cicely. Dr Cecil Williams."

It was then that Cicely realised that the Secret Police were looking for her.

She had no idea why the Kempaitai wanted her, and during the few hours before they came to arrest her she thought of the possible reasons. She had been head of the women's camp at the time of the limpet bomb episode. She had been in Singapore on parole for four months and so could have made contacts outside. She had also lived long enough in Malaya to have many friends among the Chinese and other nationalities in the country. All these things would make the Japanese suspicious, but none of them were convincing reasons for arrest and torture.

She destroyed any papers that might be compromising. There was not much. The Japanese had already searched her possessions several times and taken what they wanted.

She tried to compose herself, and thanked God that she was not liable to panic in a crisis. She tried to turn inwards and talk to herself, controlling her thoughts and feelings. It's a privilege, she told herself, and there may be much that I can do as a doctor for those who are already prisoners of the Military Police. I'm tough, she thought, I'm lucky. I have no outside responsibilities.

Deliberately she kept her thoughts away from torture and her memories from the screams she had heard from the Raffles Museum. She felt that she would not be able to stand up to torture.

Among her papers were notes on the prison diet which she had kept, hoping that they would form a valuable record as a basis for future medical papers. She found that she could concentrate her thoughts on these most marvellously. Yes, surely they would make the basis of a magnificent paper in *The Lancet* after the war. She would celebrate the occasion by inviting her friends for dinner and she would buy wonderful food and cook for them . . .

The agents of the Japanese Military Police came to arrest her at 4 p.m. on 23 October. Two military policemen went to the small area of corridor where she had her bed and curtain. They went through all her possessions and took all her papers. She never saw them again, but she managed to grab her glasses, rug and coat.

She was taken to a small office and questioned for about an hour by two Japanese. Then she was told that she would have to go to the Kempaitai Headquarters. The military police took her in a lorry to the Y.M.C.A. building.

In the Kempaitai Headquarters she was pushed into a waiting room. The first horror was the noise. All round her she could hear people screaming in torture, and during the twenty-four hours that she spent there the screaming never stopped.

The room was bare except for a table and two chairs. On the table lay a small object. Cicely recognised the rice bun she had given to Freddie not long before.

A few minutes later she was taken into the interrogation room.

CHAPTER XI

TWO MOTIONLESS JAPANESE were waiting for her, an interrogator and an interpreter. The interpreter seemed vaguely familiar. She learnt later that he was half-Malay, and had been a caddy on the Sepoy Lines golf course before the war.

The noise made by screaming victims in other parts of the building was so loud that she realised that to answer questions she would have to raise her voice. Afterwards she decided that every possible machine and every inquisitor must have been working at top pressure, not only on the Europeans and internees but also on the local people.

"Name?" The word cracked out.

With surprise she found she could answer easily.

"Age?"

"Forty-nine."

She felt that it would be no use refusing to answer, because this would only anger them. It was also no use telling lies, for she was not used to lying. She found it hard to lie or even to know what lies to tell.

"Nationality?"

She began to recognise her personal method of resistance. In Jamaica it was called "forming fool", and the principle was to go on talking, making up details and mentioning as many insignificant facts as possible, repeating lengthy descriptions and irrelevant stories simply to pass the time. Cicely had been well practised in this at school, and found that words flowed easily. It was terrifying to shout above the screams, but she felt that much of her future and indeed her survival depended on her exhausting her interrogators before they exhausted her. Obtuseness could be a useful weapon of defence.

The questioning went on and on. Where were you born? What languages do you speak? Where did you do your training?

Every detail. Oxford? Never heard of Oxford. Where is that?

"It's where your Prince Chichibu was educated." She thought this sort of irrelevant detail might help, but they said they had never heard of Prince Chichibu. She tried to make a long story of the fame and importance of Oxford and then Cambridge. Then she talked about Bath and London and Jamaica and hospitals and plantations and Africa and the sea and horses and children and examinations and lectures.

The Japanese said that a peculiar thing had happened. Whereas many men had come to lecture in the women's camp she was the only woman who had gone to lecture in the men's camp, and they thought that this was suspicious. She pointed out that permission had been obtained from the High Command in the prison. She had gone over under a Sikh guard who had been present all the time during the lectures, and had been returned to the women's quarters under the same guard. Then they asked, "What language did you lecture in?" She answered, "English."

"Why English?"

It was difficult to convince them that English was the prisoners' common language, and that in any other language it would have been impossible to convey the gist of the lecture.

"And what about this?" barked the interpreter suddenly, menacing and triumphant.

Cicely recognised the note to Professor Monro which she had given to the small boy with the twisted knee. Probably the child had dropped it somewhere, where it was picked up and handed to the High Command. It had been translated into Japanese. From the subsequent questions it seemed to Cicely that the words "*2 o'clock*" had been made into some sort of B.B.C. wavelength. They thought it was a code message. Yet in a way it was a relief to be interrogated about this because it diverted their attention, and she could discuss every detail of the child and his football accident and the whole of his past life and his future history, and this took up a great deal of time.

The interpreter was much more hostile than the inquisitor, and from time to time made gestures indicating that if she didn't answer more fully or more quickly or more sensibly she would be taken to one of the rooms where the torture was going on. Cicely was very frightened, feeling that once they started torturing her she would make up anything in the world in order to get away from it.

The inquisitor shouted in Japanese and two officers appeared and approached Cicely.

She stiffened and, expecting a blow, tried not to cower.

But they did not hit her. Instead they seized her glasses and pulled the hairpins from her hair so that it fell down her back. She started to protest in voluble English, feeling that everything depended on fighting every inch of the way and not agreeing to anything that she could possibly resist.

The officers advanced again and started to pull at her clothes. Helplessly she looked enquiringly at the interpreter.

"Elastic," he said, with a sneer. "Give them the elastic."

"But I only have elastic in my knickers," she protested, anger overcoming fear.

"Yes, knickers."

"But that's impossible," said Cicely in the shrill voice of crisis. All her power was behind her protest.

To her surprise the inquisitor muttered something and the guards fell back.

"Give them the blanket and the coat," said the interpreter angrily.

It was a steaming hot day and holding the blanket and coat close to her was unpleasant. But Cicely felt determined to keep them.

"Blanket and coat. Oh no," she pleaded. "I shall freeze without the coat. I am very old and very weak and I need them."

The interpreter translated and she saw at once that she was on a successful line. She knew that the Japanese have great respect for age. She shook her fallen hair at them, pointing out that it was streaked with grey.

"I must keep the coat and blanket. Do you understand?"

Her voice echoed her thoughts. The Japanese faltered and

moved back. The inquisitor began to look embarrassed. Eventually he held up his hand and spoke. The interpreter translated, and Cicely realised that he was changing the subject.

"Tell us again how you visited the men's camp."

Late that night they marched her to the cells. A row of cages opened on to an "L" shaped corridor, reminding Cicely of a reptile house. The entrance to each cage was a padlocked door, about 2 feet high.

As they passed down the corridor she could see people sitting in the cages. At the lower corner of the "L" a sentry unlocked the padlock on the door and opened it, motioning to Cicely to remove her sandals.

She crawled in on all fours and did not look back when she heard the small door clang behind her.

The cage was about 8 feet square with one small barred window at the back and a front of wooden bars from ceiling to floor. Inside were a Japanese soldier, two Chinese coolies and a lavatory seat. There was also a notice on the wall forbidding prisoners to walk about and stating that there must be no "membling, preaching or grooming".

Each of the four members of the cell sat in a corner. Japanese sentries walked up and down the corridor. Talking and direct communication was forbidden, but Cicely felt that her companions were friendly and courteous. After a while the guards brought little bowls of rice, but she had no appetite. During the night the Japanese soldier wanted a drink and he was given it from a bucket. But for the rest of them there was only the lavatory. Cicely spent most of the night sitting beside the seat and vomiting.

The torturers were working throughout the night. Cicely recognised the voices of some of the victims. One of them was a Chinese woman whom she knew quite well. There was no question of sleep, partly because of the noise and partly because of constant interruptions by the Japanese soldiers. At one point two soldiers came down the corridor and one started hitting the other. Cicely wasn't certain whether he was drunk or receiving legitimate punishment or whether he was still alive at the end or not. She remembered that when she was in Changi she had seen some translated documents about discipline in the Japanese Army, and one of the things it said was: "If your superior officer beats or kicks or slaps you, you must be grateful because it shows that he is taking an interest in your progress."

The cage was infested with bugs to an amazing degree. Cicely had had experience with such insects in hospitals in various parts of the world, particularly in Trengganu. But these bugs were a new experience to her, more abundant than she would have thought possible and, of course, inescapable.

Early next morning she was taken upstairs again for further interrogation. It went on all day. The questions were the same, over and over again, until she had reached a stage of exhaustion when she wasn't certain what she was making up. Again there were repeated suggestions and hints that she was going to be taken to the other department.

Late that evening she was given food and told that she was to be moved to another prison. She was taken under guard in a military lorry to a shop in Smith Street on the corner of New Bridge Road, an area of Singapore that she knew well. The ground floor had been converted into cages similar to those in the Y.M.C.A.

She was put into cell No. 5, a cage of irregular shape, about 4 feet wide at one end and 8 feet at the other. In it were seven men. They included Bill Yoxall, who had been treasurer of the men's camp, and a man in the Prison Service who had been taken in for questioning because his mattress was tied with flex wire and was therefore suspected of having something to do with a radio or transmitter. The others were four Eurasians and an aged Chinese. All of them had been imprisoned for trivial reasons.

She soon discovered that torture and interrogation went on at Smith Street as well as in the Y.M.C.A., but on the whole not at such high pressure or so continuously.

The seven men sat along the wall, cross-legged. Cicely could see from their position that they were forbidden to lean back. The sentry indicated that she should sit cross-legged just inside the door. Sitting in this position had never been her habit, and she lowered herself with difficulty. Bill Yoxall, sitting nearest to her, smiled encouragingly.

The sentry slammed and locked the door and Cicely could hear him stamping down the corridor, slapping his sword against the bars of the cages as he passed.

"It's safe now," whispered Bill Yoxall. "We're not supposed to talk, but luckily they can't hear us whisper from a distance. But don't move or even lean towards me. If they catch sight of you there's hell to pay." He smiled sadly. "I'm sorry that we can't offer you better hospitality."

"Never mind," whispered Cicely, cheerfully. "That'll keep until after the war. At least you have a vacancy for me."

There was a heavy silence and she felt that she had said the wrong thing. She could hear Yoxall breathing heavily. It was impossible to tell whether he was sobbing.

"Tell me about it," she said at last.

He shifted his position very slightly, shuffling on the floor, cocked an ear carefully to listen for a sentry, and then began to whisper.

"He was a doctor too. One of my closest friends, and one of the chief entertainers of our idle hours in Changi. His inventiveness got him into trouble. He made a mechanical clock and all kinds of other devices. He even got a sledgehammer and broke up some of the concrete couches in the middle of the cells in order to improve the amenities. The Japanese were deeply suspicious about this, and took him off to the Y.M.C.A. When he arrived here he had been so badly beaten that he could hardly walk. But this morning he was passed by the Japanese doctor as fit for torture, and they took him away. Then we heard that he managed to fling himself out of a window and died."

Again silence fell between them as a sentry walked down the corridor, turned outside the door, screamed and marched back.

"You must be careful," whispered Yoxall as soon as he had gone. "If they see you whispering they drag you out of the cage and kick you."

"I think he's coming back," whispered Cicely warningly.

"It's the one we call Fee Fi Fo Fum," said Yoxall. "I recognise his snarl."

From their cage at the far foot of the "L" they could not see round the corner, but they could hear noises down the corridor. Cicely could see into the next door cage, where the sentry stopped.

Inside there was an aged Chinese without teeth. Cicely learnt later that he had tuberculosis, was an opium addict and was in prison because he had sent money to the prisoners in Changi.

Fee Fi Fo Fum was a huge Japanese with enormous yellow boots. He dragged the old man out of his cage, held him up in the air and shook him so that his head wobbled. Cicely thought he looked rather like a minnow. He made no sound. Eventually the soldier flung him back into the cage and marched off down the corridor. For a few minutes the Chinese man lay breathless. Then he sat up and resumed his cross-legged position with an air of dignity.

"That's mild," whispered Yoxall. "A warning rather than a punishment. At breakfast time you'll see why he annoys them so much."

"Breakfast?" The word sounded odd.

"A euphemism, of course. But we do get a bowl of rice some time during the day. And from ten o'clock in the evening until seven in the morning we are allowed to lean back against each other and sleep as best we can. There's no room to lie down, of course."

"I still have my blanket and coat," whispered Cicely. "Perhaps we can all share them."

She spent the night lying flat on the hard floor. She was already stiff from having to keep a rigid position. The bright light from a bare bulb in the ceiling shone in her face, and the night seemed very long.

"Cho, cho," shouted the sentry in Japanese. "Get up." The seven men and Cicely returned to their cross-legged position. Later the guards brought small tin bowls of rice.

"Now for the music," whispered Yoxall, jerking his head towards the old Chinese in the next cage. Cicely watched carefully. The old man picked up his little bowl of rice, rose to his feet and poured it into the lavatory in the corner of the cage.

The Japanese started to scream. Cicely was not surprised for she knew that they could not tolerate this kind of scorn. Fee Fi Fo Fum came roaring down the corridor as the other guards dragged the old man out. Cicely could not bear to watch as they knocked him about and flung him on the floor repeatedly.

Presently a guard came round with a kerosene tin of tea without milk or sugar. He poured the tea into the prisoners' bowls. Both Cicely and Yoxall had bowls with holes in the bottom. Cicely tried to plug the holes with her fingers, but the tea was so hot that it burned and she only managed to drink a few drops before it all ran away. Despairingly she gazed at Yoxall, who had done no better. He jerked his head towards the corner, indicating that the only other means of quenching thirst was in the lavatory, which had to serve for drinking, washing and for the usual purpose. She wasn't surprised to learn that dysentery went constantly round and round the cages.

That day she felt that if these were the conditions under which she was expected to live she would refuse to drink, and would die of thirst rather than go on living. But when the time came she found that she could survive all sorts of things which she had never thought she could endure.

They sat in the cage for eleven days without interrogation and without a change in anybody's position. On the twelfth morning the guards came for Cicely.

In the few seconds left to her she tried to prepare herself for torture. With firm, deliberate movements she crawled through the small door and slowly put her feet into her sandals.

Along the corridor the Japanese shouted and stamped angrily. She prayed for strength.

A soldier unbolted the door at the end of the corridor. On the other side stood a forlorn figure in a tattered dress. It was Freddie Bloom.

They were marched together to the office. Behind the desk

sat a Japanese whom neither of them had seen before. After the customary pause, head bowed, he looked up and astonished them by saying in English: "I am the Welfare Officer."

Bewildered, they bowed, each wondering what was coming next.

"Since you are ladies," he said, "we have decreed that you should have special privileges. Your friends in Changi prison have sent some supplies for you which, thanks to Japanese kindness, you now receive."

Again they bowed. On the table in front of him were two bundles. He handed one to each of them to unwrap. Cicely's contained a coat and trousers, a change of underclothes and some food in tins.

"And now," he said, beaming, "you may bath and wash your clothes in the lavatory sink of the sentries!"

They bowed for the last time and were marched out, carrying their new clothes. They had to leave the food behind, and they never saw it again.

The lavatory was filthy but the water ran in the taps. They sluiced the floor and mopped up as best they could.

"Marvellous," said Cicely, squirting a jet of water across the room and letting it run through her hands. "Just to feel water, just to do something different."

"And put on different clothes."

"Best take the wet ones back with us."

"What do you think they're up to?"

Back in the reception room the place of the Welfare Officer had been taken by a fierce looking Japanese. Cicely privately christened him the Lord High Executioner. He spoke to them through an interpreter, and gave her the impression that he was high up in the Gestapo hierarchy.

Through the interpreter he told them to stand in front of him. They stood and bowed and he asked how were they? They said, Very well, thank you. He then said that the Japanese were very kind and had allowed them extra clothes. They thanked him. He said they had been allowed to wash their clothes. They thanked him again. He said, would they please give them to the sentry to hang up outside to dry. But Cicely did not trust anybody. She gave them only the underclothes and that was the last she saw of them. She tucked the frock under her arm and refused to be parted from it. During the interview the Lord High Executioner was eating pineapple chunks out of a tin with a toothpick. After he had stared at the women for some time he stuck the toothpick into a pineapple chunk and gave one to the interpreter. Then he did the same for Cicely and Freddie. At this point Cicely got the giggles but he did not seem to mind. He continued to eat pineapple chunks, ask fatuous questions, and make remarks about the extreme kindness and consideration of the Japanese Government. Eventually they were sent back to their cages.

After this the Japanese really got down to business. The first man to be taken for questioning was Yoxall. The guards came for him about eight o'clock one morning and returned him twelve hours later. They flung him on the floor and he could scarcely move. He had been beaten all over. Cicely thought that he looked like raw liver from the waist downwards.

There was little she could do. But unlike the men she had a handkerchief. All night she dipped it into the water in the lavatory and put on cold compresses. She thought that he was going to die. But next day he was taken out and given the same treatment all over again and made to kneel on pieces of firewood for hours on end with torturers jumping on his legs.

Again she tended him as best she could, overwhelmed by her helplessness and unable to control the tears running down her face. After a while he opened his eyes and said, "I earn my living with my head, not with my legs, so you needn't worry too much about them."

Cicely thought that one of the sentries on duty that night had a kinder face than some. Made bold by despair she signed to him and said, "Coppe, coppe," which means coffee.

As soon as she used the Japanese word the sentry grinned, nodded and walked away. A few minutes later he brought a tiny cup of coffee for Cicely to give to Yoxall. When he had finished it she held it out to the sentry and said Thank you, "arygato, arygato", and he brought a second cup. Then the party was interrupted by the return of two more victims of the torturers being flung into near-by cages.

It was a time of unlimited terror. Cicely prayed for death as everyone prays when they are frightened. It seemed that the Japanese were aiming at mass executions and trying to find reasons to justify them. When they found that there was little to be got from these prisoners they tried to torture people into making false statements that would justify execution.

Day after day and one by one the other men in the cage were taken out, tortured and flung back. Cicely was astonished that, out of a group of about sixty men taken from Changi who were tortured, not more than two or three broke down, and without exception they retracted under more torture. Cicely wondered when they would start on the women, and whether their holding back was the result of a pathetic wish to be regarded as civilised.

There was no food except for a tiny bowl of rice three times a day, and life was at a low ebb.

One day when things were about as bad as they could be Cicely was sitting as usual just inside the cage, trying not to be miserable. Suddenly a sentry who had been screaming and yelling and slapping his sword across the bars all day stopped his noise and stood quite still outside her cage.

"My God, what's going to happen now?" she mumbled to herself. She could not see much because they had taken her glasses.

The sentry had his hand on the top of the bar of the door, and he seemed to be signalling to her. She put out her hand, and to her astonishment he gave her a small square of plain chocolate, stamped with the familiar Cadbury tree.

"Oof," said the sentry, and put his finger on his lips.

She bit her small square of chocolate carefully into eight pieces and handed them over her shoulder to the seven men sitting behind her. All the while the sentry watched her. The next morning he came with eight squares of chocolate. She never saw him again.

She did not think that Yoxall would survive. At one time the doctor gave orders that he should be taken to hospital and have both his legs amputated. Then the message came back that there was no room in the hospital.

The Japanese seemed to resent Cicely trying to help him. On 9 November they came to the cage and told her that she was to go to another cage. Now she could only leave him her blanket, her hope and her admiration.

She was moved from cell 5 to cell 4, six foot square, containing a lavatory seat, three men and herself. Again there was not space for all to lie down. But at least there was no bright light. It had gone wrong and no one had bothered to fix it.

Cicely knew that she was replacing a man who had died in that cage a couple of days before as a result of torture. One of the remaining men, Cyril Jackson, had been through the same torture as Yoxall and more. It was now three days since his last interrogation. He was in severe pain. He was allowed to remain lying down most of the day. In the morning when the sentries came and said, "Cho, cho!", meaning, "Get up, get up!", the others would point to Cyril Jackson and say that it was impossible. Some of the sentries spoke a few words of Malay, and prisoners could communicate with them a little. It wasn't until ten o'clock at night that they came round and screamed "Yasumi!", and then the prisoners were allowed to lie down. Two people could lie and one curl up in the corner. The fourth had to sit up.

To Cicely the redeeming feature of the small cage was that everyone was considerate, even though they sat still all day long and were not allowed to speak. During the daytime the sentries were very alert. But after the guard had said, "Yasumi" she heard a tiny voice behind her from Cyril Jackson, saying, "Miss Williams, would you like to do your toilet?" This courtesy from this bleeding wreck was an example of the way she found that people behaved under such conditions. While she did her toilet the men turned their backs. Sometimes the sentries would come and take an interest in it, but then the men would rise to their feet with unanimity to protect the lady's toilet from the sentries' gaze.

She managed to keep her sarong, and this was enormously useful. Yoxall had her blanket, Cyril Jackson her coat, and the sarong was a protection for her toilet. She also wrapped it round the tummies of people who got dysentery one after the other. She used to sit on it when she had developed a floor sore from sitting on the hard ground with no protective fat on her behind. When the mosquitoes were bad they would stand up and flap the sarong about. The mosquitoes became particularly troublesome when the Japanese ran out of the oil which kept them under control.

They were not allowed any implements. The men were not allowed to shave or have their hair cut. They bit their fingernails to keep them under control. But they could not bite their toenails, and these became increasingly uncomfortable. One day one of the men spoke up gallantly.

"I'm going to give you one of my trouser buttons. I think that you can use it for sawing the edge of your toenail and then peeling off the rest."

She found that this worked. Then someone tore a sliver of wood from the floor which they could use as a toothpick, and this too was a great comfort.

"One thing I have learnt," she whispered one night when the sentries were less vigilant than usual. "The minimum essential equipment for cagelife is a toothpick and a trouser button."

For two years after she came out of prison, she carried these two things wrapped in a small piece of paper stuck inside her clothes. It was only when she found that she was no longer carrying them that she felt emancipated.

The men's hair and beards grew down to their shoulders. Their moustaches grew uncomfortably into their mouths. Cicely made some pomade with grains of rice to wax their moustaches. All her hairpins had been taken away, and she could only comb her hair with her hands.

One of the diversions in this cage was two cockroaches. They called them Gert and Daise, and cultivated them as part of their morning routine. Every morning the creatures used to walk down from somewhere in the roof, stand on the bars and wave their feelers at the prisoners. But then they became impertinent and tried to eat the rice sticking out of the men's moustaches, so they had to be liquidated.

Sometimes they were given a little toilet paper. They used it for paper-folding games. On Cicely's sarong there was a criss-cross pattern. They made draughtsmen out of round and square bits of paper, and played draughts whenever they could do so without being caught by the guards. Sometimes in the afternoon the guards were slack and they could lie down. Then the door at the end of the passage would suddenly open and the guards would try to catch them out. The pounding on the floor as all the men tried to get up quickly always reminded Cicely of big dogs scrambling to their feet at the sound of riding boots on the stairs. In the evening when the guards were slack they would talk softly and tell stories.

But during the time when the sentries were most strict they were not allowed to talk at all, though they did communicate with each other. Some knew deaf language, finger talking. As they sat on the floor they would write letters and spell out words which the others could see. At night they told endless stories, discussed every aspect of the situation and their home lives. They recited poetry and sang songs in a sort of *sotto voce*. To Cicely's surprise and comfort, in this group there was never any competition for food or other unpleasantness.

2 December was Cicely's fiftieth birthday. That morning the guard on duty was a young Chinese conscript whom they called Yo. His real name was something else, but this was the Japanese name for a conscript. When Yo came round with the tea he slipped a tiny parcel to Cicely. It was about one inch square, and he said in Malay, "Birthday, other Mem". Freddie Bloom in a near-by cage had remembered her birthday and had somehow got hold of a piece of soap which she had sent as a birthday present. Cicely returned it to her next day because it was very precious.

Freddie was in a larger cage which also contained fifteen

men. Among them was Walter Curtis, a devout Catholic of immense Christian fortitude and patience, who had managed to send his wife and six children to Australia before the capture of Singapore. He had been brought up in Japan, and could speak Japanese as well as English. He was constantly being called on by the Japanese to interpret, and because of his gentle manner he was able to get all sorts of information and various concessions from time to time. When the sentries roared up and down the corridor Walter Curtis would stand at the bars of his cage, bowing to them and making polite noises in Japanese. And after speaking to them for some time in this manner he might be granted a concession; perhaps somebody would be allowed to lie down or they would bring extra tea for somebody. It was through him that Freddie had been able to get the piece of soap.

When Cicely and Freddie were interviewed by the Lord High Executioner he told them that they could come every day to have a bath in the sentries' washroom. After this they were allowed out occasionally, perhaps once or twice a week, at irregular intervals.

"It seems to me that they only allow us here when they want the place cleaned up," said Freddie. The sentries' lavatory was always filthy.

"It makes a change," said Cicely, squirting water from the tap.

"Well, when people talk about the Japanese being such clean little people they obviously know different Japanese from ours."

"But even so you can have a much more satisfactory wash here than in the lavatory seats in the cages," said Cicely. "And it's nice to have a bit of gossip."

She particularly appreciated this because it was Freddie who usually provided the gossip. There was more traffic in her cage than in Cicely's. Men came and went from different prisons, and Walter Curtis sometimes got information from the Japanese guards.

At one of these meetings Freddie said to Cicely, "Wonderful news. Walter has persuaded the Japanese to give us privileges at Christmas. We can say our prayers at midnight and sit up until that time."

It was a small excitement that gave hope unrelated to religious beliefs.

But at ten o'clock on Christmas Eve they were ordered, as usual, to lie down rigidly on the ground. Midnight came, but no permission to get up and say their prayers. Cicely lay awake, listening to everyone else lying awake. The clock struck one, then two. Sentries shouted and stamped in the distance and an eerie depression settled over the cage. Cicely found it impossible to stifle her deep sense of hopelessness.

The clock began to strike three. She was now longing for sleep.

Then the door opened.

"Cho, cho," shouted the sentry.

They soon realised what had happened. Ever since the Japanese took over they had been on Tokyo time, three hours ahead of Singapore time. The sentry had decided that they would prefer to say their prayers by their own time.

On Christmas morning each prisoner received a slice of sweetened rice bread and some rice wine. They celebrated again at New Year. The Japanese made much of this festival, and told them they would have a wonderful time. This consisted of being given a minute tot of something called "stag whisky", made locally and tasting so. They were also given a sort of purple bean curd and told that it was a Japanese delicacy. Cicely felt that at least it was a gesture of goodwill.

"It's delicious," she said, and meant it. She had calculated that at that time their average diet was not more than 600 calories a day. They were all weak and emaciated, and beginning to show signs of beri-beri, with septic sores. Cicely had a whitlow on her finger which she concealed as far as possible because she did not wish to have treatment from the so-called doctor, who she felt was merely a toady to torturers. She hid it under her handkerchief, but one day a guard noticed it and told her that she had to be examined. Several sentries watched, and the medical orderly indicated that he proposed to pull off the nail. He produced an enormous pair of forceps. Cicely refused, categorically, which made all the sentries roar with laughter. Then the orderly said he would incise it. She allowed him to do this, and was pleasantly surprised at his skill and the sharpness of his knife. He then applied the smallest dressing that Cicely had ever seen, and she realised that he must have been taught specifically how to economise in dressings. In the New Year she developed impetigo, which caused much pain.

Traffic in the prison was brisk. Many people were taken for examination and never seen again, and one day Cicely's cage was emptied and she was put into the large cage with Freddie Bloom. She was delighted to be with Freddie, but found conditions in this cage more trying than in the small one where all had been friends and considerate to each other. Here people were breaking up into groups and competing. Some were desperate, some dying, and some so miserable that they didn't bother about anyone any more. It seemed to Cicely that the atmosphere was approaching the lowest stages of animal life. But there was one big compensation: they were allowed to take a little exercise for a few minutes after meals. The cage was about seventeen feet long, and with the greatest pleasure Cicely would walk from one end to the other, trying to walk along one line of the floorboards.

By this time many of the men had dermatitis and a sort of pellagra of the scrotum which made it painful to sit down. Some had torn the pockets from their shorts to make small jock straps. All were in rags. The slacks which had been sent in to Cicely from the camp were worn through in the seat. Freddie managed to get hold of a piece of handkerchief. Walter Curtis, their great standby, managed to borrow a needle and thread from the Japanese, and Freddie sewed a patch on to the seat of Cicely's trousers. Walter also managed to get back her glasses. Because the Japanese had respect for him he was allowed to have a Testament, and it was the first time Cicely had read anything for three months. A Sikh in the cage had been allowed to keep his comb and sometimes he lent it to the two women, which they felt was a very great privilege.

Across the corridor was another big cage. Talking was severely restricted, but Freddie devised ways of communicating with the people in it. As they sat on the floor they would spell out letters on their knees, looking into space as they did so. Or they would talk to each other in deaf language. Freddie and Cicely recited poetry to each other and translated nursery rhymes into French. Devices of this sort kept some sort of mental activity going, but they were all becoming weak and mental processes were slow. The days were long and somnolent and the nights long and sleepless. For hours they would sit doing nothing, and sometimes Cicely would resent Freddie trying to start off mental activity, thinking to herself, "Can't she see I'm busy thinking?"

When she managed to sleep she had marvellous dreams, usually of gardens better than any florist's catalogue, and of the countryside and rooms of big houses and social events, all of a fairylike quality. In one dream she went into a room which had been furnished as a landscape, with rocks made from grey velvet and a stream running through it with the most superb flowers and trees and shrubs.

The most unpleasant part of their hunger was still the perpetual mental preoccupation with food. It was impossible to speak or think or read without thoughts of food dominating the mind. Cicely managed to convince herself that what she ate was enough for her, and this helped a good deal.

Every ten days or so the Japanese would produce a handful of salt for the cageful of prisoners. This aroused deep feelings because some of the men craved for it. They developed a strict ceremony for its distribution. Cicely had to go and stand in a corner and hide her eyes, and each man placed a sheet of lavatory paper on the floor, making two rows. Each knew his own piece. Then Cicely would divide out the salt in little equal piles, and there was trouble if they weren't exactly equal. Most of the men kept their store and just had a tiny taste from time to time.

The Chinese New Year was in February, and by this time their old Chinese friend was in the big cage with them. The

Japanese had tried every brutality to get him to confess what he had been doing and with whom. Having failed, they changed their tactics and treated him better than anyone else. They took him out and gave him a superb Chinese New Year's feast, hoping that this treatment would induce him to give away his information. But after this first decent meal for months he crawled back through the door into the cage, spitting blood, and said, "These rotten people, they had any amount of food, why couldn't they give it to us all?" His antagonism was unchanged.

They had bad dysentery in this cell. It went round and round, for there was only one lavatory between seventeen, and this was also their only source of water. Walter Curtis made strong representations, but nothing happened.

One day a sentry brought a small pile of spinach, and told Cicely and Freddie to go to the courtyard to make a fire and cook it. They asked for some oil and, to their surprise, it came. The spinach ceremony was repeated on a number of occasions, and Cicely was amazed to see how quickly people's health improved when they were eating the green vegetable. She also much enjoyed being called out to help with the cooking. At the end of the courtyard there was a gate with big bars which was not entirely blocked from the street. A sentry usually stood there, but occasionally it was unguarded. One day Cicely was stirring the spinach in the pot when she heard a voice calling out through the gate.

"Missie, Dokitah, Tabeh!" She looked up in astonishment, but no one was there and no one called again. She decided that it must have been one of the amahs from the Hospital who saw and recognised her but darted out of the way as quickly as possible in case some sentry heard. Cicely was much cheered to hear this voice from the outside world.

One man died of dysentery and others were very sick. Eventually they managed to persuade the Japanese to let them have some buckets of water that did not come from the lavatory, and also a cup.

Freddie was swelling from beri-beri, and could no longer

wear her slacks. She had to wear Cicely's sarong instead. By begging the Japanese they managed to get a bottle of yeast tablets to keep her going.

On one of their occasional visits to the sentries' lavatory Freddie became excited.

"Look," she said, pointing to the floor. "Newspaper."

Some of the previous visitors to the lavatory had evidently used it, and there were still some scraps on the floor, which they salvaged and washed under the tap. One fragment was from *The Singapore Times*, now under Japanese control and called the *Shyonan Shimbun*,* but still in English.

From this scrap of paper Cicely and Freddie learnt that the Allies had attacked Monte Cassino.

But where was Monte Cassino? No one in the cage knew. The words became a sort of question mark over the cage for many weeks.

About two months later things began to change. First the men were allowed to shave. Then Cicely was given scissors and allowed to cut their hair. A few days later they were all called up to the office. Some of the men and Freddie were told that they would be discharged and sent back to the camp. Cicely was told that she was not discharged but was temporarily to be allowed back in Changi prison. The feeling that it was temporary haunted her for the rest of the time before they were liberated. She was never certain that she would not be taken back to the Kempaitai.

Later that day a lorry arrived and took them back to Changi prison. It was March 25th, and they had been under the Kempaitai for over five months.

* *Shyonan* means Rising Sun and *Shimbun* means News.

CHAPTER XII

"What heaven to be back!" Freddie said this more seriously than she intended, and gazed up at the concrete walls of Changi prison. She was swollen with beri-beri and found it difficult to control her legs. Cicely tottered beside her weak but not swollen.

No one had heard anything about them since they were taken away five months previously. There was great rejoicing that they were alive. They were given a room together in the sick bay, and extra food. Cicely's first horror was sleeping in a bed after so long on the floor. All night she kept finding her arms round the legs of the bed, terrified, and certain that she would fall.

There was news to catch up with, some of it grim.

"John Long was executed."

"Is Norman Coulson still as helpful in getting things for us?"

"He died. They couldn't find an excuse for executing him, so they starved him to death. That's happened to many people."

They were kept in hospital for a week. Later Cicely realised that no one, including themselves, had any idea what sort of time they had been through or how low they were in health. As a result Freddie did not get good treatment for her beri-beri, and was sick for many months.

"Something's afoot. We're going to move."

"Repatriated?" This hope was in everyone's mind so the rumour swept through the camp, neither confirmed nor denied. Since the Double Tenth no one had been allowed a newspaper, not even the *Shyonan Shimbun*.

One day Miss Simmonds came hurrying along the corridor in such excitement that it seemed she must have news.

"Look," she cried, and shook an object at them. It was Cicely's trousers.

It was the pair that Cicely had worn in the Kempaitai. They were blue, and the patch that Freddie had sewn on was a piece of a red and white handkerchief, which Miss Simmonds had thought indecent. An industrious member of the sewing group, she had taken them away and now returned them with a fine patch of strong black material, spade-shaped and no less conspicious.

Cicely leant forward to thank her, but a woman at the back forestalled her by giggling.

"The arse of spades?"

A flush appeared on Miss Simmonds' cheek. It was the only time Cicely ever saw her angry. Without speaking she rolled up the slacks, tucked them under her arm and hurried down the corridor. Cicely never saw them again, but a few days later she gave her a beautiful pair of black silk amah's trousers. Cicely hated to think how much sugar ration or rice she must have sacrificed to get them.

The rumour about moving turned out to be true, but there was no question of repatriation. They heard that they would be moved out of Changi prison to Sime Road, which was an old R.A.F. camp with hutments. And a great move it was.

"I'm astonished at the possessions of people who have nothing," said one of the men sent over to help the women move. At that moment he was carrying a rusty bucket filled with dry earth. The earth was dropping out of the bottom. To the handle of the bucket was tied a string, and to the string was tied a brick. All this was part of the precious belongings of some wretched internee.

"Everyone has collected things," said Cicely, "although we have practically nothing and have been given very little." She was looking at a small pile of tins, bits of string, nails, pieces of paper with recipes, Italian lessons and history classes.

"Isn't it wonderful to get away from the concrete and the walls?" cried Katherine de Moubray. At Sime Road Cicely was sharing a section of hut 1 with Katherine, Freddie and another woman.

"Look," cried Freddie. "Ronald Searle! I recognise his drawings, and here's his signature. He must have been a prisoner here with the R.A.F."

All round the walls were frescoes of prisoners and chickens and officers in ragged uniforms. And food and cooks in kitchens, and still more food.

"Wonderful commentaries of life here when it was a military prison camp," said Cicely admiringly. She felt cheered and excited by the new experience.

Food became even scarcer. The daily rations were a little soft-boiled rice with some kind of spinach. Very few of the Red Cross parcels ever reached the internees. Smoking anything that could be smoked became a common habit.

"Should one smoke the Gospels? It seems a terrible thing to do."

It was a Sunday morning, and Cicely was playing bridge with some nursing sisters. Tobacco arrived regularly, though without paper. Occasionally the Japanese gave out piles of old newspapers which were supposed to be used for other purposes, and they made bad cigarette paper. Recently the prisoners had been given a stack of pamphlets written in Chinese on paper which smoked quite well. Now someone had discoverd that it was the Gospels.

"It's written in Chinese, so I don't see that it really matters," said Cicely, who had given up smoking at the beginning of her imprisonment in order to trade her tobacco ration for other needs.

"I've already begun to smoke my Shakespeare," said one of the sisters.

"Oh, that's terrible," said her partner. "Fancy smoking Shakespeare."

"Well, I don't really think I shall miss *Timon of Athens*."

"Listen," called Cicely.

They heard a strange new sound, a growing roar. They ran out excitedly. Overhead aeroplanes of a type that they had never seen before gleamed silver with swept-back wings and dropped bombs on Singapore. The four women watched with apprehension, awe and joy. It was the first sign of Allied activity they had seen since February 1942 and this was 5 November 1944.

"Aren't they wonderful!" said one of the sisters, starstruck.

"Can't we find out what's going on?"

They were still allowed no newspapers. Sometimes a kindly Chinese passer-by would wrap one up in a stone and fling it over the wall. Sometimes the men who went out of camp on fatigues would collect news. A secret radio was still operating in the camp, but it was controlled by a close society and the women could not get any B.B.C. news. Rumours increased, but months passed. There were occasional raids, but still no reliable information. They had heard something vague about D-day, and when the first atomic bomb was dropped on Hiroshima a Japanese sentry told one of the men prisoners that a peculiar and extraordinary bomb had been dropped, but no one knew what this meant.

Cicely's health was deteriorating again when, during the early months of 1945, military prisoners were brought over to dig trenches outside the women's huts.

"What are those for?" asked a naïve young nurse. But there was no need to answer. Everyone sensed that the Japanese planned to liquidate the prisoners if they were conquered.

One of these long trenches was just behind Cicely's hut. As her illness developed so the desire increased to grow something edible outside the window. So far she had been too weak to dig. But now she got some sticks of cassava, broke them across her knee and walked along the top of the trench, sticking in pieces at intervals. It was only a gesture, but to her surprise it grew fast and better than anyone else's.

Soon after this she found that she could no longer walk. She struggled for some weeks, but had to give in and spent more than a month lying in the camp sick bay.

She came out of hospital just after VE day, feeling for the first time that there might now be hope. Just over the barbed wire from her hut men were digging foxholes and trenches. The Japanese were using both military and civilian prisoners, and urging them relentlessly to work. The men who came to dig were not allowed to look at the women or speak to them, and if they did they were kicked and hit by the guards.

One day Cicely watched from the window as three soldiers of the Argyll and Sutherland Highlanders arrived under Japanese guard. Instead of getting down to work one of the men waved his hand and shouted to the women on the other side of the barbed wire. He seemed to be ignoring the Japanese guards close by him.

"My God," she said to a woman standing near her. "That man's mad. They'll shoot him."

But still the soldier waved and shouted. "Girls. Have you heard? It's going to be over. They're going to sign on the dotted line." He turned round to the Japanese sentry and said in Malay, "Isn't that true?"

Cicely was astonished to see that instead of kicking him the sentry took off his hat and grinned and bowed. She thought, the world has gone mad.

At a committee meeting later that day she asked if anyone had heard anything and no one had. They must be mad, she thought again, and there the matter rested in her mind.

But two weeks later she was sent over to the men's camp in charge of some women and children who were going to see doctors. When she arrived a man hurried up and said, "Come quickly and see what has happened." He took her into one of the huts and there, to Cicely's astonishment, was a creature who looked like a god. He was dressed in a camouflaged coat with a little red beret. He was a doctor, and had dropped by parachute that morning.

In theory they weren't kept in any longer. Yet it seemed strange to Cicely how little this, or indeed the whole business of victory, eased their lives. The doctor had asked about stretcher cases so that arrangements could be made to take them away: yet many days later these patients were still there. He had also asked what they needed most, and they had told him bully beef and letters. Again for weeks nothing happened, and then the R.A.F. started dropping lipstick and knitting wool.

"Peace comes dropping slow," said Freddie, sighing. But she had at last heard that her husband was alive in a military prison.

But there were new anxieties for Cicely.

"We must try to restrain the young people," she said. "The Japanese may still shoot us all if they lose their tempers." The older women went round and talked to the younger.

"For God's sake show them that you can take it coming and going. Show them that we're used to winning as well as losing. Bite your tongue and don't change your behaviour one inch. Go on bowing and carry on exactly the same."

One morning Cicely heard a shout over the barbed wire.

"Cicely, Cicely. Come!"

It was Dr Leo da Silva, a pathologist. He was not a first generation Eurasian and had not been interned, but had worked at Tan Tock Seng Hospital all the time.

"I can't," said Cicely, suddenly immobilised and full of fear. "What do you expect me to do?"

"Come," he said, encouragingly. "Climb over this gate. I'm going to take you out and give you lunch."

"I can't come like this." She was suddenly ashamed that she wore no shoes or stockings. Even her sandals were now worn out. She had only a sun top and khaki shorts.

"Oh yes, you can. Get over this barbed wire. I have a car."

Lunch! A car! It seemed impossible. But somehow she climbed the wire. He put her in the car and told her that it ran on rubber spirit. Soon she was in Tan Tock Seng Hospital, sitting on a chair at a table while he opened a tin of Heinz mushroom soup.

She felt a strong desire to lick the plate and kept saying to herself, No, no, you mustn't. You'll never get used to civilised life again if you do. It was an achievement not to lick, and she felt proud.

Later that day her boy Ali, whom she had not seen for four years, came to see her. He had heard that she was in camp. He said that he wanted to wash her clothes and clean her house. Her "house" was a space 4 feet by 6 feet on the verandah of the hut, and her clothes were a couple of pairs of khaki shorts and a sun top. Later Ali came back with his wife Mina, but by this time Cicely was feeling ill because she was developing malaria. Late in the evening she again heard Ali's little pattering footsteps. Mina had gone home and cried because Cicely was so thin, and she had made Ali put all the family dinner into a tiffin carrier, curry and some rice and bananas. And after that he came every day and swept out Cicely's 4 feet by 6 feet. Before she got on the ship to go home to England he came with three dozen fresh eggs which she put in a tin and took with her. In England in 1945 the sight of so many eggs was sensational.

From then on people began to visit them and bring food. Then Mountbatten arrived and the troops marched into the camp with a military band. Most of the women cried, even those who had controlled themselves for years.

The troops didn't like the smell of the women, and this was not because of dirt, for by now they were all clean. Cicely decided that it was what people talked about in Africans, the point being that if people are on a different diet they smell different. Starving people smell different from those who are well fed.

The first member of Mountbatten's staff she met was Jack Scharff, from Trengganu. He came to the camp to find her. He had a car and took her to Changi prison, where the military were interned. He wanted to go round the wards and meet some of the doctors. Cicely took the opportunity to question him. At first he was reticent, but she was persistent and calm.

"When are they going to give us jobs to do?" she asked. "There's so much to be done."

He hesitated. "As a matter of fact, Cicely, it's all arranged."

She chose to ignore the embarrassment in his voice. "When do we start and where?"

"Mountbatten has brought in an administrative staff."

"You mean new people?" She could hardly believe it.

"New to Singapore, yes."

"But he can't do that," she cried. "They don't know what's been going on. They won't know what's needed. We're the ones who know."

"Yes, Cicely, put like that you're right. But," he hesitated, "you're all in bad health. You need leave and rest."

"Well, only briefly," she said with determination. "We only need a little food and we'll be all right. There's so much to be done that we ought to start right away."

By this time she could see that something was amiss, and she probed deeper.

"Well, as a matter of fact," he said reluctantly at last, "we didn't expect to find any of you alive." He told her that they had been certain that the prisoners would all be dead, for they knew that the Japanese planned to put them down if they had to surrender. The atom bomb had saved them. The Japanese felt that this was something with which they could not be expected to compete, and so they could surrender without losing face.

"I don't know who these new people are, but I think it's most unwise," said Cicely, furiously. "We, who know this country, should stay now. I'm going back to Trengganu."

"I'm afraid there's no possibility of that," said Scharff. "The ships that brought out Mountbatten's troops will take you back to England."

"I won't agree," she said petulantly. "I'm going to a higher authority."

He sighed. "The next person above me is Sir Ralph Hone, Chief Civil Affairs Officer for Malaya."

She went to see Sir Ralph and the interview was brief.

"There's no question about it," he said. "If you refuse to go you will be put in irons and put on the ship."

"All right," said Cicely. "I'll go to Mountbatten."

But that night she was in bed with a temperature of 103° and malaria, and in no condition to argue.

A few days later, still weak and feverish, she was on a Dutch ship bound for England.

The day before she left she was told that Mountbatten would

take the surrender of the six Japanese generals, and Lady Mountbatten wanted six women from the camp to be a sort of guard of honour. Cicely went, wrapped oddly in a huge white coat. Lady Mountbatten sent a car to take her to the house where she was staying with her staff. Cicely found that she was scared of them, so polished and enamelled. She felt anxious trying to sit in a chair and drink the cup of coffee that Lady Mountbatten gave her. During the ceremony they stood on a balcony overhead, high up outside the High Court, with a panoramic view of the ceremony. Cicely was terrified. The troops were keeping the lines, but when the Japanese arrived she thought the people in the crowd were going to break out and savage the Japanese. She found the animal noises made by the large crowd of people longing for revenge unbearable, and she thought, "My God, there are going to be more horrors now." But nothing untoward occurred.

The ship gave them small appetising meals without second helpings. Cicely was impressed at the foresight of the authorities, for when the prisoners had first been freed some of the men had insisted on going into Singapore and had died from overeating. She knew that this happened easily after starvation.

Many of the Dutchmen on board had relatives in Indonesia, including the Captain, who had heard nothing of his wife and children for four years. But instead of going on to Indonesia he had to turn back and bring the prisoners home. It was an unhappy ship. There was still much anxiety for many people. Even for those whose main anxieties were ended it was a period of strange adjustments. They sat about on the decks listlessly and refused to wear their new shoes or sit on chairs. Cicely was surprised how impossible it was to feel free or hopeful. Many of them felt worse than they had felt in prison. "We're never going to be fit for anything," Cicely thought in her gloomiest moments.

"What is the matter with us all?" she asked one of the military doctors.

"Not much," he said, reassuringly. "We were briefed about you before we left. Apparently ex-prisoners have a curious outlook and mentality for a while. That's all. You'll get over it."

They called at Colombo, and the ships in the harbour were dressed to welcome them. When they landed they found that the ladies of Colombo had prepared huts for their comfort. Cicely knew that they must have been short of clothes themselves, but everything that could be spared had been put into these rooms, including magazines and books. There were bowls of fruit and places where they could wash their hair. There was mail, too, but Cicely was too upset to read hers, even the telegram. She stuffed it in her shirt unopened.

They were each given £1 to spend in Colombo, and she went out with two friends to wander in the town. Presently an English girl came up and said, "Are you booked for lunch? My parents would like you to come and the car is here to take you."

To Cicely's surprise the car was Government House's largest. The girl was Miss Monck-Mason Moore, the daughter of the Governor, and a medical student.

The three of them, dressed no longer in their rags but in comparative elegance, thanks to the ladies of Ceylon, climbed into the Governor's car.

"I feel like Queen Alexandra on Rose Day," said Cicely, looking out on the crowded streets where people were bowing and waving to them as they passed. But the only thing she could think of buying was a pair of sandals.

They drove to Government House. On the doorstep stood an A.D.C. in uniform with frogs and gold lace.

"Isn't he gorgeous?" whispered Cicely to her companions. "I'd forgotten that people could look like that."

He greeted them as though they were normal people and said, "Luncheon will be at one o'clock. Perhaps you would like to have a rest and a bath beforehand?" They were shown into three enormous bedrooms, each with a marble bathroom. But it was too much for them and they ran from room to room in fear. Then they wallowed in the baths and put on some of the clothes they had been handed in the ladies' huts. At one o'clock they were summoned to cocktails with His Excellency before luncheon.

"Tell us about some of your experiences," said a woman brightly, as though asking them to describe a holiday. The gulf between them widened beyond communication. Cicely could only mutter incongruously.

"We aren't really fit for human company."

"Nonsense," said the woman, briskly, but not unkindly, and started to ask tentative questions. Had the Japanese behaved unspeakably? How much had they had to eat? Was it true that some people had escaped? They tried to shield her from the horrors yet still to entertain her. Cicely thought they weren't doing too badly.

But suddenly the woman turned away and started to talk to a friend. Cicely overheard her speak in a high distinct voice.

"Why on earth does the old man insist on having these poor jailbirds here? It's ghastly for us having to listen to their stories."

Shocked, Cicely stared across the harbour. In a subtle way she felt more deeply and treacherously wounded than at any time during her imprisonment.

"Look," said the Governor, coming through the door with his guests. "The ships are saluting you."

There was noise and disturbance. The ships in the harbour dipped their flags and blew V-signs on their hooters. Bands were playing. Everyone began to cheer and clap, and suddenly Cicely was aware of the future emerging from the past.

CHAPTER XIII

As soon as Cicely was healthy again she went back to Malaya to be in charge of all Maternity and Child Welfare services. This was the first superscale post in the Colonial Service ever given to a woman, and the first of a series of important appointments. She was now fifty-two, and still had nearly a quarter of a century of working life ahead of her. Her ideas were formed; future years would enrich but not change them.

She now had knowledge that was strong and enduring because it was supported by experience and feeling. She knew that the future of any country or community lay in its children, and that the confidence of parents in the survival of their children was of first importance. She knew that this confidence could only be based on personal responsibility, but as long as children's deaths were commonplace few parents could feel this confidence or sense of responsibility. Instead they would tend to be fatalistic, often attributing such deaths to the will of Allah, the evil eye or some hostile spirit.

Moreover, the conditions and diseases that kill babies and children damage others. Where many die, many others survive maimed or sick. So, contrary to common belief and official practice, she was convinced that the basis of a community's health lay in its maternal and child health services. All over the world these must be developed if health was to improve.

In undeveloped countries, where people died young, as many as eighty per cent of the people were women and children. Yet nearly all the health services and nearly all the hospital beds were for men, always more powerful and vociferous.

By the time she left Malaya three years later Cicely had formed the strongest ideas about medical services in developing countries, about feeding the world's children and about the control of population that was beginning to become so important. Over the years she found herself increasingly at variance with official views on these subjects. She became convinced that the Western world was wasting opportunities and vast sums of money by tackling these problems in the wrong way, trying to provide food and other materials that were lacking, instead of dealing with people at an individual level and by education.

After a period at Oxford she joined the World Health Organisation, and was soon Advisor in Maternal and Child Health, with South-East Asia as her parish. After leaving W.H.O. several years later she worked in Jamaica, then in London, but continued to make frequent journeys abroad, for the University, W.H.O., or as a Nuffield visitor. Always she fought her battle, at times, it seemed, almost single-handed, against tropical malnutrition. One day she added up her travels, and found that during her life she had worked in fifty-eight different countries. She had become one of the most remarkable doctors of our time, and gradually her influence increased across the world.

In 1960 she went to Beirut as Professor of Maternal and Child Health in the American University, and she stayed there for four years. At the age of seventy she returned to London, and became adviser in overseas training to the Family Planning Association. Having spent her working life making the world safe for babies, she ended it in trying to make the world safe from babies. The difference to her was not so great, for the most important aspect of both, she was convinced, is the proper care of mothers and young children. Only when life is safe for babies and where children are healthy and parents confident will people voluntarily limit their families. It is no use trying to arrange it the other way round. Reduction of quantity is not possible until good quality is assured, and it is a waste of time to introduce family planning methods without also doing everything possible to ensure the survival and good health of the children who are born.

Increasingly, Cicely Williams' message is preached, and her methods practised, in tropical countries everywhere.